NURSING INTUITION

HOW TO TRUST YOUR GUT, SAVE YOUR SANITY, AND SURVIVE YOUR NURSING CAREER.

JENNIFER JOHNSON
BScN RN

First published by Whimsical & Enchanted Stories 2024

Copyright © 2024 by Jennifer A Johnson RN

All rights reserved. No part of this publication may be reproduced, stored or transmitted in any form or by any means, electronic, mechanical, photocopying, recording, scanning, or otherwise without written permission from the publisher. It is illegal to copy this book, post it to a website, or distribute it by any other means without permission.

This work, including all written content, narratives, and accounts of lived nursing experiences, is protected by copyright law. No part of this publication may be reproduced, distributed, or transmitted in any form or by any means, including photocopying, recording, or other electronic or mechanical methods, without the prior written permission of the copyright holder, except in the case of brief quotations embodied in critical reviews and certain other non-commercial uses permitted by copyright law.

Disclaimer: The opinions and views in this book are mine and have no reflection on any past or present employer. The events are how I recall them. Names are never included unless with consent, and neither are timelines. I will always do what is best for my patient and all details have been changed to protect every aspect of anonymity. Dates, times, places, and distinguishing features have all been changed. Any seeming connection to real time and place events or people is purely coincidental.

Jennifer A Johnson RN has no responsibility for the persistence or accuracy of URLs for external or third-party Internet Websites referred to in this publication and does not guarantee that any content on such Websites is, or will remain, accurate or appropriate.

For permission requests, please contact Jennifer Johnson at jennjohnson222@gmail.com

DEDICATION

I dedicate this book to my family but specifically to the backbone of who I am—my mom and dad. You put up with my crazy schedules and ups and downs. I hope this book helps you to understand why I was as kookie as I was. Thank you for your support and for the understanding, care and compassion you extended towards me and my journey. I love you more than you could ever know.

To Trevor. You thought you were marrying one person and ended up with an upgrade (but very different wife) by the time this book was finished. Thank you for your support and love through all the absolute best (and worst) moments. I know you've heard these stories time and time again. Thank you for being my rock – and letting me make you more into a crystal.

To my children, Wyatt, and Elise. I love you with all my heart and soul. Everything I do is based on something that reminds me of you! Know that I'll always be with you, even if I'm not.

To my hundreds of co-workers. You're all MVP's. I've watched you grow and am so proud of the nurses and people you've become. We're family. That's all there is to it. Special mention to my work wives —you know who you are.

"One day you will tell your story of how you overcame what you went through and it will be someone else's survival guide."
—Brené Brown

TABLE OF CONTENTS

Preface 7
Introduction 8
  1 | The Game 11
  2 | What is that Gut Feeling? 15
  3 | What Intuition Feels Like 23
  4 | Empathy: The Core Nursing Value 27
  5 | Think Critically 33
  6 | Violence and Safety 37
  7 | The Importance of Calm 43
  8 | Medical with a Sprinkle of Magical 49
  9 | How to Protect Your Energy 55
10 | Intuition Story Time 61
11 | Caregiver Fatigue and Moral Distress 63
12 | Exercises for Resilience 71
13 | Habits and Rituals 79
14 | Nursing Specialties and Their Abilities 83
15 | A Day in the Life 85
16 | So, Your Patient Has Died 93
17 | Shadow Work 105
18 | Self-Care Routine 111
19 | The Toxic Co-Worker 117
20 | The Most Toxic Place I've Ever Worked 121
21 | My Introduction to Nursing 131
22 | Bully Encounter #2 135

23 | Bully Encounter #3 139
24 | Showing Up to a New Unit 149
25 | A Note About COVID-19 153
26 | The Final Straw 157
27 | How to Survive Nightshifts 161
28 | Will 165
29 | Ghost Stories 169
30 | My Best Story 173
31 | Emotional Resilience 179
32 | An Ending or A Beginning? 185
Appendix | My ER Pump-Up Playlist 187
Glossary 189
Endnotes 191

PREFACE

THIS IS A COLLECTION of my lived experiences—skills acquired, lessons learned, and traumas felt. They are written as I remember them. Some stories are new; others have been waiting to be told for over a decade. I share these stories for learning purposes. As you read them, take what resonates, and (if nothing else) know that nursing is quite hard and we're all struggling. You are not alone.

Looking back, I wish I'd had advance knowledge of what my nursing career would be like. I still would have continued in nursing as I *love* my job. I just don't love some of the lasting marks it's left— mentally, physically, and spiritually. Remember, we're all in this crazy thing called nursing together, and it's a family regardless of where your home base is.

The work will always be there. People get sick and require care, but if you don't take care of yourself first, you may not be there to provide the help needed. Do you treat your patients the way you treat yourself? I'm guessing the answer is no. None of us would leave a patient hungry, not showered for days, teeth unbrushed, and sitting in dirty clothes. You would never leave a patient in physical pain. Don't leave yourself in a place of emotional pain. It's time to give yourself permission to look inward. You deserve a chance to heal, too. How are you going to move forward? Do you continue with the status quo, or are you going to choose *you* today?

If you're looking for a sign, this is it.

INTRODUCTION

THANK YOU for picking up this book! This work was written in six weeks, born in a sleep-deprived state as a trauma journal. To be truthful, other than getting up super early and staying up long after everyone else was in bed, I don't recall much about writing it. It began as a way to process the pain, stress, and anxiety of COVID-19, and a way to explain to my children (if I died) why I decided to continue to work in the ER during a pandemic.

Things took a severe right turn to include "intuition" once I put together that all the stories I had written down. At the same time, I knew I couldn't possibly use that word in a book without peer-reviewed, scholarly articles behind it. So, that's what I went searching for. Lo and behold, there's not just an abundance of science supporting the notion of intuition, but specifically intuition in nursing practice.

As you read *Nursing Intuition*, I want you to try and put yourself in my shoes. As I work through the case studies and exercises, I want you to do the same. Write in the book. Mark it up. Burn it at the end if need be. But, put your soul into it as I have. I know you've felt your gut scream at you, but have you listened?

Use this book how you need to. If you want to jump from chapter to chapter, or go in sequence, it's up to you. The first few chapters describe the science behind intuition and then the book transitions into my trauma journal entries, and more than likely yours will as well.

If you need a secondary journal for writing space, feel free! There should be enough room provided within these pages for you to stop, in the moment, and write down whatever comes up for you. An intuition exercise within an intuition exercise if you will. However, if you find that one topic is too much to be able to move on from, then I suggest you stick with it until you feel like you've purged your heart and soul onto the page. Follow your gut, even if it sucks, there is a reason for it.

No matter what, please know that you are not alone in your struggles and suffering within nursing.

Reach out for help if you need to because we are not meant to do this alone. We are nurses. We are stronger together, and we need to begin to help ourselves as much, if not more, than we help others.

In Canada and the USA:
If you or someone you know is thinking about suicide, call or text 9-8-8. Help is available 24 hours a day, 7 days a week.

1 | THE GAME

IT BEGAN as a simple game, both to kill time and amuse myself while I worked triage for twelve straight hours. Many of my co-workers refer to triage as *story time*. It's someone's first contact with nursing staff as they come into the ER. They sit in pain, scared, worried and running worst-case scenarios through their head while they wait to be triaged.

People don't usually come to the ER unless they are in a fair amount of pain or have been told by a friend or relative (sometimes medical, sometimes not) that they should *get that checked out*. They arrive, sit in close quarters and wait for their turn to see the nurse for assessment.

At triage, we classify people from sickest to those who can wait. This determines how fast they will see the doctor. Most people who come to the hospital assume that they are the sickest one there, or are in the most pain and should be seen the fastest. Sometimes they believe they will be seen in the order they arrived but the emergency department is *not* urgent care. The difference being urgent care doesn't provide access to life saving interventions and is only open during business hours. Sometimes people get confused on this point.

Anyways, it was a game. A game I was good at.

I'd look at someone walking through the door and guess why they were coming in. I would look for cues as to what was happening—were they holding their stomach or chest? Were they obviously bleeding, or did they just look unwell? I would make my predictions based upon what I thought was happening and then wait until they came into my triage booth to ask, what brought them to the emergency room that day. The number of times I was close to the right answer grew. I was getting good at the game and I was addicted to playing it.

Over the years, I got better at the game and as a result, upped the stakes. I made my guesses more specific—from abdominal pain to gallbladder issues to appendicitis. Once the person got in the triage booth, it was my job to figure out roughly what was going on so I could place them within the department. I aimed to be accurate with how sick they were, figure out their path through the emergency department, determine the amount of nursing care they needed, what lab work and medical directive would follow, how quickly they needed medications and then, finally, receive their assessment by the doctor or nurse practitioner.

Some cases were easy to predict. Most people were straightforward with their complaints: a laceration is a laceration; a broken arm is a broken arm. But, at least once a shift, someone would come in and my gut would scream that there was more going on—that something much deeper and more concerning was happening, even though the evidence didn't suggest it. Something was wrong, and I knew it. Even though I didn't know *how* I knew it. Having a standard complaint or their vitals looking good didn't change how I felt. *Something* was wrong.

Perhaps the person had good vital signs, and yet their *color* was off. From pale to grey to green tinged, something about their color cued me to the fact that something more was going on. It was those people I would check in on through their journey within the ER. Half of my concern was to make sure that their condition wasn't deteriorating. The other half was to see if my gut instinct was right. Occasionally I was wrong, and the doctor would give me a funny look regarding my over-concern, but I was usually *right*. The person often deteriorated quickly but, thankfully, we would already have this patient in the right area of the ER with their lab work done and the doctor already having seen them with further diagnostics completed (CT and/or X-rays).

This game became kind of an obsession. The more I listened to my gut, the more often I was right! It was a mix of experience, knowledge, and gut instinct that made me a great triage nurse. When I finally started to talk to other nurses about my game, they said they either did it as well, or were going to start. Talking to other nurses about their experiences with their gut instincts and their internal "knowing" when something was off was freeing! I wasn't nuts! I wasn't alone in feeling what I felt. I began to understand just how powerful this was when it came to taking the best care of my patients.

Assessing how I "feel" about the patient's condition is now a conscious part of the assessment of my patients whether I'm in triage or working in a part of the ER. Do I think they're improving? Are the current treatments improving the presenting illness and symptoms? Do I think this patient will harm me? Am I at risk of violence? Will this person give me trouble— either medically or behaviorally? Am I seeing their vitals trend in the wrong direction? Does their plan of care need to change? Do I think I will need the doctor with this patient later in the shift?

These are the questions I began asking myself for each of my patients at the beginning of my shift, and I recommend you do, too. Some of your answers will be guided by the report you receive from your colleagues going off shift. Experience will also play a role, but listen if your gut feels heavy or if you get bad *vibes* about a patient. By conducting your assessment with *all* your senses and not just the physical picture, you can discern more about your patient. Nursing knowledge is achieved through empirical, aesthetic, personal, and ethical knowing, while intuition is demonstrated through the *art of nursing*.

CASE STUDY

Paramedics brough an elderly lady into the ER after she was found at the bottom of a set of steep stairs in her home. EMS stated that she fell after missing the last step and was unable to get up. When asked how long she had been on the floor, EMS said they weren't sure. I went to assess the patient and saw the slight outline of a woman on the stretcher, covered in a dark grey sheet from EMS.

She was a bit bruised and a little cool to the touch. Her pale, thin skin let the icy blue of her tiny veins peek through. She seemed well enough, but my gut told me different. She was breathing on her own, small little breaths that barely moved her chest. Her vital signs were stable, but something told me there was more was going on than what I was seeing in front of me.

Within our medical directives, I ordered basic bloodwork, but because of how I *felt*, I added on a CK (creatine kinase – a marker of muscle breakdown, something we don't normally order). Knowing the emergency doctors I routinely worked with, gave me a bit of leeway when ordering more tests than are included in the medical directive.

Around thirty minutes later, the doctor came around the desk and asked who had ordered the CK. I felt sheepish as I had not worked with that specific doctor before but said "I'm so sorry, but I did." The doctor proceeded to thank me, saying that he would not have normally ordered that bloodwork. It showed that her CK was extremely elevated and was now in a rhabdomyolysis.

Rhabdomyolysis is a condition where the muscle breaks down and leaks CK into the bloodstream. This can do a lot of damage to the kidneys if the patient isn't over-hydrated with IV fluids to flush out the excess CK. If Rhabdomyolysis is left untreated, severe kidney damage can happen and may lead to kidney failure. However, because I had ordered the CK, we were able to avoid it and save her kidneys.

I was shocked. I ordered the CK after hearing that the patient was on the floor of her home for an unknown amount of time. I remembered hearing that this could cause muscle breakdown and then an elevated CK. To this day, I can't differentiate between whether it was my gut, or unconscious knowledge that inspired my decision. Truly, it didn't matter. What mattered was that the patient's kidneys were spared because we caught the problem early enough and were able to treat it appropriately. It was a win.

I didn't care at the time how I knew what to do. I just trusted that there was a reason it popped into my head when it did. I am so thankful I went with my gut because it turned out the patient was the mother of a prominent doctor who had retired from the same department years prior. This had no bearing on the treatment of the patient, but the son of the patient was very thankful I had gone above and beyond to care for his mother.

This is how it started. I began to listen to the things that "popped "into my head, seemingly out of nowhere. I started paying attention to my gut when something felt off or didn't add up. Most important of all, I stopped questioning *how* I knew what I knew and, instead, started to lean into what my gut was telling me, trusting it more with each win.

When I say intuition, what's the first thing that comes to mind? Start putting a bit more belief in the things that pop into your head when you first ask the question.

It's time to learn to trust your gut!

2 | WHAT IS THAT GUT FEELING?

INTUITION is defined by Merriam-Webster's Dictionary as "the power or faculty of attaining direct knowledge or cognition without evident rational thought and inference." Many other descriptions of intuition have included a heaviness in the gut, a feeling of just knowing something was *off*. Your breath quickens, you get goosebumps, (or as I like to call them *truth-bumps*), a shiver runs down your spine or your heart suddenly races. For me, intuition feels like a heaviness in my gut and a sense of just "knowing." When I'm on the right track, I get goosebumps all over my forearms. This signifies to me that I have either said something or had a thought that needs more of my attention.

Intuition is also defined as presence, with clear insight. In other words, it is a human ability for knowing or doing without adequate reasons, and is a way to recognize truths without rational thinking. Intuition is that intangible thing that many experienced nurses rely on without realizing they are doing it. It's a niggling voice in the back of your head saying that you need to be careful in a certain situation, look closer or reassess your patient. If you feel comfortable talking about this with a nursing friend or if the topic comes up on the floor in conversation, pay attention to those who know *exactly* to what you are referring. Ask them for examples and what they did in those instances. Listen and learn from other people's experiences.

Many experienced nurses know this feeling well and have integrated it into their practice without even realizing it. An example is the nurse who, when they give you handover on a patient (or transfer of accountability), tells you "I don't have a good feeling about this...keep an eye out." That will be the patient they ask you about the next day to see how the night went. They will want to check to see if their gut instinct was right. Talk to these experienced nurses and ask them *"why?"*! Why were you so concerned about the patient? Was there a lab value that did not sit right with you? Can you explain what that felt like? When did you feel that about the patient?

They may not be able to give you a lot of answers. No one has likely ever asked them about what they've been feeling and why. Try not to be upset if they can't give you any specifics. They may come back to you after a day or two wondering why you were asking those questions. You could give them a variety of answers or simply say that you happened to either hear about nursing intuition or were reading a book about it.

Since the 1980's, there have been countless studies about nursing intuition and how it's an untapped resource. Unfortunately, back then, we didn't have the ability to test those theories. With ever-changing landscapes, advances in technology and simple interest in the field, breakthroughs have finally happened. "Intuition has a basis in both tacit and formal knowledge. Tacit knowledge is seen as implicit knowledge that is obtained by experience in the field, while formal knowledge is the knowledge gained by training and education." In more recent times, there have been advances in brain imaging that have led to testing hypothesis in intuition and the subtle physical changes it can produce. "Electrophysiological studies confirmed the existence of intuition and proved its emanation from the frontal cortex of the brain. In this case, the brain and heart have an interactional relationship for receiving, processing, and decoding the intuitive messages." With these advances in medical science, we can further prove—not only the existence of intuition, but start to figure out a better way to cultivate the feelings.

THE ART OF NURSING

For all the focus on evidence-based practice and the push to continue to update our knowledge on any given topic in nursing, there is a subtle undertone of the "art of nursing." While it follows evidence-based practice, it also acknowledges that working with people and dealing with life and death situations results in occurrences that we cannot understand or comprehend (yet).

I was truly fortunate in my nursing education to have the core value of *trusting your gut* be in the forefront of the conversation. If it wasn't the teacher in my lecture bringing up the subject, it was discussed by the clinical instructors or nurses we were paired with for clinical placements. At the time, it seemed to be more of an *unspoken* rule. Since they couldn't prove a link between nursing intuitive concerns and evidence-based practices meant it was sometimes talked about only in hushed tones.

It's within the idea of science meeting spirituality that *Nursing Intuition* was born. There is evidence that the intuitive system is an indispensable element for health professionals' decision-making. The intuitive system, is not necessarily less capable. On the contrary, complex cognitive operations eventually migrate from the rational system to the intuitive system (i.e., they become more automatic) as capacity and skills are accumulated.

In the emergency departments where I've worked, nurses will have the occasional conversation about a patient. We chat about our concerns and why we're not sure they will do well. If I voice my concerns to my doctor, the supportive doctors will, at the very least, ask me why. If I say I don't know, they tend not to push me further but usually go and take a second look at the patient. That is all I ask.

I am incredibly lucky to have worked with many supportive doctors who don't bat an eye when I ask them to reassess a patient. Inevitably though, you will be met with a sneer from someone who doesn't understand what you are saying. Usually, these doctors are the younger medical residents who have not had the experience, or opportunity to feel the intuition for themselves. After this happens, they start to listen. They may even wonder what they may have missed in earlier assessments, growing their own intuition as a result.

CASE STUDY

This case happened when I was a new graduate in an exceedingly small, rural hospital in a town of less than 5,000 people. We didn't have access to CT scans or specialists. It was usually just the emergency doctor who was also the family medicine doctor providing care to the people of the town.

NURSING INTUITION

I was in my unit listening to a taped report (I'm talking cassette and recorder.) about a patient who had a history of alcohol abuse and chronic pancreatitis. Nothing in the report was overly pressing and no new concerns were present, as the patient had already been in the hospital for a few days. I walked down a short, sparse hallway to room three. There, in the second bed closest to the window, was my patient. The man looked much older than his stated age. His leathery skin spoke to a life spent outdoors in the sun. His vital signs were within normal range, but before I could get deep into my assessment, he doubled over in pain—grabbing at his abdomen, and crying out. I quickly rechecked his vitals and found that, unexpectedly, everything was slightly out of range and quite abnormal. His heart rate and respiration-rate had jumped up and his blood pressure had started to drop. The man seemed to be in agony, holding his abdomen and rocking side to side. I called his doctor who was not yet in the hospital. She answered, sounding a little like I had just woken her up.

"Yes" she piped out, sounding more than slightly aggravated.

"Hi, it's Jenn. So sorry to call you," I said somewhat sheepishly, "but your patient in room three who was admitted with pancreatitis isn't doing well. I saw him at 8 a.m. and now he's doubled over in agony. His vitals are all over the place, and I don't know what to do."

"It's okay. What was his lipase (a bloodwork value that reflects if there has been damage to the pancreas) this morning?" she asked. I provided her with what seemed to be an alarmingly high lipase. "Okay, he's been admitted before, with his lipase higher than that, so don't worry. I'll be in when I can," she said. Before I could answer and continue to voice my concern, she hung up.

I sighed to myself. "Well, if she's not that concerned, then maybe I'm overreacting."

I left the tiny, oblong nursing station with its glassed-in area and returned to room three to reassess my patient. My mood was sour. Being hung up on didn't seem very professional, and it just didn't sit well with me. My patient continued to roll side-to-side in a rhythm of agony, his pain-stricken face looking even more pale than before. I kept the vital signs machine at his bedside with the blood pressure cycling every five minutes. His blood pressure continued to dip, his heart rate and respiration rate slowly increased and beads of sweat appeared on his forehead.

2 | WHAT IS THAT GUT FEELING?

I *knew* something was off, but what?

Satisfied after my reassessment that something was very wrong, I made sure to have fluids running through the intravenous as fast as they had been ordered as I waited for the doctor to arrive. I gave the patient what pain medications I could, being very cautious of the amount in relation to his blood pressure, and the effect they could have on it.

Nervously, I paced up and down the short hallway, continually checking to see if the doctor had arrived. It was only thirty minutes that went by, but in my mind, it felt like an eternity. I had continued to repeat vitals, and a concerning trend became evident: his heart rate and respiration-rate continued to increase while, ever so slowly, his blood pressure continued to fall. At the time of the doctor's arrival, the vital signs were not terribly abnormal. Blood pressure was in a normal range even though the patient had been hypertensive throughout the night.

I pressed the doctor to see the patient however she continued to brush me off in favor of reviewing the bloodwork. Another forty-five minutes passed before the doctor finally saw the patient. She agreed that he seemed to be in pain and blamed the changes in vital signs on that. More pain medications were given while the doctor completed her assessment. It was at this time I felt that I finally had a minute to assess my other patients.

Another forty-five minutes later, I once again made my way to room three. My patient was no longer writhing in pain. He seemed more comfortable and was laying back in the bed. However, I noticed that his color was off, and his abdomen was quite distended. Once again, I repeated his vitals and the trend continued of high heart rate, lowering blood pressure, with his temperature now starting to climb. His abdomen was quite distended—rounded, taut, and firm—a change from his earlier condition. In fact, this was a significant change from his abdomen earlier in the morning and, again, my gut *screamed* at me that there was more going on than what was being seen at face value.

I went to seek out the doctor who was reassessing her other patients on the teeny, tiny medical floor. I mentioned the changes in his abdomen, and the continuing trend of his vitals. "Oh, good, that means his pain is better managed," she replied. "The pain medication is causing him to relax, and that's what's causing the drop in blood pressure."

"Oh," I say, "but what about his heart-rate and his temperature rising?"

"Just run the fluid bolus that I ordered, and that should help," she said, turning away from me, seemingly to end the conversation.

In that moment I felt two feet tall and utterly defeated. What else could I do? I had repeatedly brought up my concerns, only to be cast aside. I felt that because I was a brand-new nurse, I was not being taken seriously. I felt so disrespected. To be treated that way after doing what I thought was my job was an awful feeling.

With very few new orders to process for my patient, I was forced to sit and wait and watch. His color got worse – it went from deathly pale to pale grey to a grey-green undertone. His vitals continued to become more unstable and he developed a full-blown fever of 101.3°F. His abdomen also continued to become firmer and rounder. It was around eleven in the morning when the doctor finally decided to reassess the patient. It was only then that she finally felt that something wasn't right.

We moved him into room five, our one cardiac room. It was a private room, rarely used and usually only when there wasn't room elsewhere on the floor to put a patient. He started to become less responsive, only occasionally opening his eyes when we put him on monitors or started another IV. We repeated bloodwork, then IV fluid boluses were started just as his pressure was dipping into the low 80 mmHG's systolic. He became less and less responsive as the minutes progressed. Within the hour, we were running both levophed and dopamine (inotropic agents used to keep up blood pressure). These were our last lines of defense to keep his blood pressure above 70mmHG systolic. He had stopped responding to us, and the treatments that we had started. Ultrasound wasn't available as it was a Saturday. We had called the X-ray technician in to do an ultrasound and X-ray, but they weren't in the hospital yet. Bloodwork was repeated, and it wasn't looking good.

By noon, we were doing compressions as his heart had stopped. Code Blue was called overhead, and the few other staff in the hospital came to help. It felt like round after round of CPR was administered. It was another 45 min before he was pronounced dead, and we pulled the white linen sheet over his body. The doctor called his family and tried to explain what had happened.

I was shell shocked.

2 | WHAT IS THAT GUT FEELING?

Things had happened so quickly. I was *so angry* that the doctor hadn't listened when I first expressed my concern. All I could do was chart to cover myself and continue with the day as I still had other patients to attend.

Later that day, we prepped his body for the morgue after the little bit of family he had said their goodbyes. I watched as the family filed down the hall, entered room five, and surrounded him. And wailed. I think they were caught off guard. It was all I could do not to break down into tears of frustration as they came to thank me for all I'd done. What did I do? Could I have done more? Should I have pushed harder? Could I have changed his outcome? I was going crazy with the "what ifs."

It was five agonizing years before I ever got any sort of validation for my efforts that day. I'd finally quit that job, and was about to move eighteen hours away to a brand-new start to my career. It was only *then* that the same doctor told me to trust my gut. She told me to not let anyone tell me I didn't know what I was doing.

Looking back, even if the doctor had listened to me, I don't know if it would have made a difference. We were in a remote, northwestern Ontario location, and I don't truly know if we would have even been able to get him out to a bigger hospital in time. All that matters now, is that I've learned to stand my ground, watch for a change in the patient's status, and trust myself when I feel something is off. It was a *big* nursing life lesson, that's for sure.

After that incident, I decided to pursue as many certificates in nursing as I could get my hands on. I knew that one day I would be leaving that hospital and wanted to be the most educated nurse to ever quit that place.

When you think about your gut feeling – what are the sensations that come to mind? It's time to start taking stock of when it happens.

Take the first step.

3 | WHAT INTUITION FEELS LIKE

INTUITION can feel like a lot of different things all at once. Someone may say something, or you could be assessing your patient and suddenly, a *feeling* hits you that something isn't right. It may come over you like a cramp or heaviness in your stomach. It could feel like there's another voice in your head telling you to look again and reassess, because something feels off. Maybe you just *know* that the outcome for a patient is not going to be good— without having a lot of supporting evidence for that conclusion. Some get a flash of a scene in their mind of something happening to the patient, or it could be that you can "smell" death. (I'm not sure if everyone can smell death or just a portion of us.)

In the summers between university semesters, I worked as a personal support worker in a long-term care facility in my hometown. It paid better than a Canadian Tire job and was closer to my career end goal of becoming a nurse. I provided hands-on care to people and it gave me a *much* better understanding of how hard personal support workers and healthcare aides work.

I would show up to work, walk through the door, and a smell like damp moss mixed with something acrid would hit me. It's still difficult to describe but when I smelled that smell, I would think *who died?* or *who was dying?* Nine times out of ten, I was right. One of our residents would have died the night before. I never gave it much thought until I talked to people in nursing school who had yet to work somewhere where death could happen at any moment. When I mentioned "the smell," I would get funny looks, and be asked what I was talking about. But sometimes, someone else who had been in those situations would join in and agree, saying, "you know, the *smell*." It was the smell of death. A smell that experience and my own intuition could identify.

I think about the conversations I've had with different nurses through the years. If I heard someone mention that they didn't think something was going the right way, or they felt off about a patient, I would strike up a conversation. It was an opening to ask my questions:

- "Why don't you think this is going the right way?"
- "What makes you think something bad is going to happen?"
- "What do you think is behind that gut feeling?"
- "When that feeling hit, where did you feel it?"
- "What did you feel when you got the idea that something was going to happen to the patient?"
- "Do you feel it in your gut? Is it a knowing? Or do you picture something happening?"

It turns out that everyone is different in how they feel/experience their own intuition. Most say they feel it as a heaviness in their gut. This is how I feel it. I often wonder if this is because there was such a strong, quiet emphasis on *following your gut* in nursing school. I wonder if I feel it this way because that was the way I anticipated the feeling to come.

EXERCISE: FINDING INTUITION AROUND YOU

Ask how people at work feel about their gut instincts.

Listen to what your colleagues say, while also noticing the language they use to describe it.

Ask and listen and then *Learn* from other's experiences.

Be mindful that asking these questions may be triggering for some people. Intuition experiences are not always positive. Watch for expressions of guilt, shame, and feelings of regret and then support your fellow nurse through this! Let them know that they still learned a valuable lesson (however hard) through this experience. Ask them what they learned and how their practice has changed since the experience!

You may notice that some nurses (and other medical professionals) are anxious and overly concerned about specific diagnoses or symptoms. This may seem odd to you or minor in detail. I would bet that the individual(s) had an experience where they missed something, or something happened that changed their practice. My anxiousness emerges related to charting, (I was chewed out by a previous manager for lack of charting when a physical page of my charting went missing, and the patient complained about my care afterwards) pancreatitis (see Chapter 2), bullying (this could fill an entire book) and ectopic pregnancies (I almost had someone bleed out on me and die).

These are things I harp on because my previous experiences have colored and changed the way I practice. I try to share my stories with other nurses so they can learn from my mistakes. Some are eager to listen, some try to listen, and others roll their eyes and walk away. All these reactions are fine because their experience will be different from mine. I choose to try and help people avoid my past pitfalls but whether or not they listen is up to them. I just hope they never end up where I've been when things go south.

When was the last time someone seemed over cautious about something that seemed minor to you? Or is there a symptom or medical condition that immediately has your back up?

Ask questions and learn from the multitude of talent that surrounds you.

4 | EMPATHY: THE CORE NURSING VALUE

HAVE YOU heard about empathy? It is "fundamental to therapeutic communication and integral to quality patient care." Many nurses that I've talked to have described feelings of empathy without directly calling it by name. They say that they can "understand where the patient or family member's frustration or anger is coming from." It usually happens after an incident that is highly emotionally charged.

Empathy is the ability to understand and experience other people's feelings and can be divided into three components: the sharing of a patient's emotional state; the explicit understanding of a patient's emotional state; and the prosocial behaviors that follow.

What many do not seem to realize is that, while many nurses are, or can have, moments of empathy, some of us will physically *feel* the feelings of another in moments of highly charged emotions.

"Nurses who possess a sufficient level of emotional intelligence are well placed to provide services in a way that improves patient satisfaction. They tend to understand interpersonal messages better, have better listening skills, and demonstrate more insight than their counterparts without such capabilities."

Have you noticed times when you were feeling perfectly calm one minute and then, after an emotionally heavy encounter, you feel overwhelmed with the exact same emotion the patient or family member had just been displaying? Do you catch yourself getting really upset, angry, or frustrated after dealing with an extraordinarily tough patient or family member? If so, you may be an empath. Empaths are people who not only understand why someone is upset. Empaths also experience a change in the way they are feeling. In high tension moments like a resuscitation or a new cancer diagnosis, we see how the patient reacts and it affects us more than we would typically like.

Do you come home after a taxing day at work and feel beyond overwhelmed? Unable to settle down? Depressed or sad with no real reason? Do you find yourself purposefully trying to *zone out* with either the TV, your phone, alcohol, or other substances (legal or otherwise), just to get the weight of the emotions off you?

If you are feeling called out, I'm sorry. To be fair, this is very much my experience as well. When I first started nursing, I would describe it as picking up a little black cloud. For almost two years, I would cry every day after work. I was overwhelmed, stressed out, and worried that I was going to do something to lose my license or worse – hurt someone with my inexperience. There's more to this story, but we'll get there in a little bit.

Normally, being overly empathetic wouldn't be such a dreadful thing.

For example, if a friend isn't acting like themselves, you'd feel that something isn't right and would ask them about it—making you a more caring friend, someone who listens and is in tune with what is going on around them. The problem comes when you are working a busy nursing job, that (potentially) has you interacting with twenty-five or more patients (and family members) a shift. These same patients are looking to you for support and encouragement. That is *a lo*t of emotion and expectations from *a lot* of people. This becomes even more overwhelming if you are new to the profession or working in a new area. You are potentially taking home more of your patients' concerns, worries, and emotions, than you realize.

If this resonates with you, and you're an empath, then congratulations! However, before you Google-search the crap out of this title, let me tell you some things.

First, it's not as much of a negative quality as some people would have you believe. It's a bit of a *superpower* in the way that you can quickly distinguish and read a situation that you've just come upon. In the emergency room, many of my patients lie to me at some point during my assessment. For example, how much they've had to drink, versus how they got their presenting injury. Everyone lies. Usually, it's not that big of a deal but, in some situations, it can change the way I triage and how quickly they get seen. Being an empath helps me see through the deceptions.

4 | EMPATHY: THE CORE NURSING VALUE

Empathy can be exhausting, but there is hope. Identify situations that can be triggering for you. Consider how how someone else's emotions affected you.

- How did you feel before versus after the interaction?
- Was there a significant shift in how you were feeling?
- Did the situation leave you drained?
- Did *your* behaviour change due to someone else's reactions?

The next time this happens, you will be more aware of what is happening. When you feel the emotions rising – and notice yours changing too – take a *breath*! If it's safe for you and the patient to do so, step away and collect yourself. Recognize that you are being triggered. Being aware is half the battle. Awareness allows you to change your reaction. Stay calm. Taking slow, intentional breaths will help.

Once you are out of the situation, reflect, reflect, reflect! Getting a handle on the types of emotions that affect you the most, will lead to finding activities that help you to manage your reaction and your own emotions. Try keeping a journal of these interactions; the emotions involved, your reactions and the reactions of others. This will help you to identify patterns of behaviour and what your triggers tend to be.

CASE STUDY

The police escorted a transwoman patient who was in their custody into our ER. One officer was male, the other female. The male officer was being unnecessarily loud and obnoxious when it came to dealing with this (also) very loud patient. The two of them were egging each other on, as the male officer continued to deadname the patient, which was obviously very upsetting for her. The officer clearly wasn't helping the situation so I kindly asked him to step out of the patient's visual field while the female officer stayed in the room. It took several minutes to calm the patient down to get to the root of her anxiety; the police had confiscated her vaginal dilators.

She stated that she had recently had her bottom surgery for gender reassignment and needed to dilate frequently to prevent her new vaginal vault from collapsing.

In talking with the police officers, they admitted that they had confiscated the dilators at the time of arrest. The patient was adamant that all she wanted to do was use the dilators to preserve her recent surgery. In speaking with police, my charge nurse, and my doctor, she was cleared to use the dilators if one hand remained cuffed. The female police officer and I were present to make sure the patient continued to be safe. We also made sure the patient didn't insert or remove anything from her vagina that could later be used as a weapon. The patient was able to use her dilators and was extremely thankful.

In speaking with the male officer after this incident, it was clear he didn't understand what being transgendered meant and that, maybe, he didn't even truly believe it was something that people experienced. After talking with him at length, I was able to get him to understand that the patient had been waiting (her whole life) to be in the body she felt she was supposed to be in since birth. It was only after the surgery that she was able to experience that. In the end, the patient was released to the police. The female officer still interacted with her most, as it was clear the male police officer was uncomfortable with the situation.

Before leaving, the male police officer asked me if I ever considered a career in hostage negotiation as he felt I was a natural. It was one of those moments where I felt I was exactly where I was supposed to be at the right time. Providing education and advocating for LGBTQIA+ community was a win that day. I'd like to hope, at the bare minimum, that the officer walked away with a bit more compassion, empathy and understanding of the trans community and the LGBTQIA+ community as a whole. To this day, that interaction is a highlight of my career. I felt in my bones that I had made a difference.

4 | EMPATHY: THE CORE NURSING VALUE

JOURNAL PROMPTS

When was the last time you had a win?
_____
_____
_____
_____

What was the situation?
_____
_____
_____
_____

Was it your patient or someone else's patient that you were helping?
_____
_____
_____
_____

How did you feel?
_____
_____
_____
_____

What did you learn?
_____
_____
_____
_____

NURSING INTUITION

Did you trust your gut?
_____
_____
_____
_____

How did you celebrate?
_____
_____
_____
_____

If it was *almost* a win, was there something you would have changed or done differently about the situation?
_____
_____
_____
_____

Did you reach out for help?
_____
_____

Was it your win or a team effort?
_____
_____
_____
_____

When you notice someone else having a win, remind them to celebrate! Praise them for a job well done. Sometimes, in nursing, the compliments and "wins" feel few and far between.

Make sure to celebrate each other!

5 | THINK CRITICALLY

MY DAD has a saying that I frequently heard growing up. "Can't you see the potential for disaster?" he would say, matter-of-factly. I'm sure it started out as a way to get us kids to think about the potential harmful situation we were about to put ourselves in, but it's also an incredibly useful saying when it comes to nursing.

In nursing school, we were told to think critically, but no one ever told us *how* to do it. Using my dad's mantra turned into an effortless way to adopt a framework of critical thinking. For example, what happens when I give a blood pressure medication but have not checked the patient's blood pressure? Worst case scenario is I drop their blood pressure so low that I must then give them fluids and potentially other medication to keep their blood pressure up. This would likely have a negative impact on their hospital stay and their health, and I would have made a medication error that could potentially seriously harm someone. Easy answer? Think ahead. Take the blood pressure *before* you give the antihypertensive medication. If you are concerned about how low the blood pressure is, *hold* the medication and talk to a senior nurse or the patient's doctor about adding parameters to the medication order.

Planning for, and anticipating, serious negative outcomes can save you from hurting someone. It can also save you a lot of work, fear, guilt, and repercussions from work due to your actions. This is the core understanding about the concept of critical thinking – plan for the worst outcomes by either preparing for them or performing actions beforehand to avoid the poor outcome before it has a chance to occur.

The most common examples that I have encountered, are listed below:

Action: Giving blood pressure medications.

Risk: Lowers blood pressure to a point where you must stop everything you are doing and intervene.

Think Critically: Take the blood pressure before you give these types of medications. This also applies to taking heartrates and some blood pressure medications/heart-rate medications.

Action: Reporting a heart rate is elevated above 100 beats a min and/or blood pressure is low.

Risk: Putting the patient into fluid overload.

Think Critically: Check that the cuff is placed appropriately and is the right size for the patient. An overly large blood pressure cuff can give you a false low pressure. Recheck the blood pressure once more and, for assurance's sake, check the other arm as well. If still elevated, expect the doctor to order a 500 to 1000 ml bolus of Normal Saline (NS) or Lactated Ringers (RL). Does the patient have congestive heart failure, swollen legs or is swollen all over? Maybe run the bolus over an hour or two instead of over 30 min. Once the bolus is finished, reassess the patient and their vitals.

Action: Assisting the patient in getting out of bed for the first time since they were admitted to hospital.

Risk: Patient could get dizzy, could be too weak to stand, or could fall and incur more injuries.

Think Critically: Get a second pair of hands to assist. Sit the patient up slowly. Are they dizzy sitting up? Have them dangle their legs over the side of the bed. Are they strong enough to stand? Let them try to stand. Do they put all their weight on you? Are they able to pivot or take a step? Always be careful as you never know someone's baseline status with mobility.

Action: Putting in a foley catheter.

Risk: Urinary tract infection if not done under sterile conditions.

Think Critically: Always have a second catheter ready and with you. Gather everything you need *before* you start including lube, (lots of lube) especially lidocaine lube for men. This will make your life easier. Have the call button within reach of your elbow or give it to the patient if they can follow commands and call for help if needed. Open kit before pulling patient pants/briefs down. You can always wear a pair of regular gloves *under* the sterile gloves if they're clean, that way, once the sterile part of the procedure is done, you can take the dirty gloves off and have clean gloves on underneath, ready to go.

Action: Organizing your day—speaking with the doctor.

Risk: Missing your chance to talk to the doctor because you were busy somewhere else or unprepared for the conversation. This results in callbacks—wasting your time and theirs.

Think Critically: At shift change when you are getting transfer of accountability (TOA), ask if there are any medication orders or consults that need ordered or clarified. Make a list of your concerns for the doctor at the beginning of shift. Leave the list on the front of the chart in case you miss the doctor. (This obviously works better for dayshift than nightshift, but if nightshift does this and dayshift does not, the note will still be there for the doctor when they get there.)

Action: Knowing each of your patient's code status (Full code or Do Not Resuscitate).

Risk: Not knowing or not clarifying a patient's code status means that you would normally treat each patient like a full code. This means you could potentially run a code on someone who wished to die peacefully without intervention. If they are resuscitated and put on a ventilator when that was against their wishes, the family are now the ones to decide to withdraw care and remove the endotracheal tube rather than the patient. This ends up causing not only physical pain for the patient but emotional pain and suffering for the family.

Think Critically: Get the doctor to clarify the patient's wishes *in writing*. If this has not been addressed, it should (at least) start the conversation and get the patient thinking about their wishes. They may also want to include talks with the family so that *everyone* knows the patient's wishes. This is my most critical point because, if someone indicates a desire to die comfortably, I am *not* going to be the nurse who accidently resuscitates them.

Action: Putting yourself into a potentially unsafe situation.

Risk: Injury to yourself depending on the type of violence i.e. verbal, physical, emotional, or sexual. Emotional risk to the patient as well.

Think Critically: Never put yourself in a room with a closed door if you have any hesitation about the other person in the room with you. Always have an escape plan when working with potentially violent patients. When it comes to the care of violent patients, the key is to be calm, cool, and collected and try not to react if provoked. The less you react, the clearer you can think about the whole situation including their care. Sometimes, this lesson takes a while to learn. In nursing, we are often required to treat "confused" patients who are not in their right mind due to drugs, alcohol, or other substances. The threat of physical violence has somehow become part of our job, and our exposure to violence is staggering. This can create emotional trauma and possibly physical injury as well. "There are more reported incidents of violence against nurses in Canada than firefighters and police officers combined."

> *Put yourself first and foremost when it comes to your safety.*

6 | VIOLENCE AND SAFETY

Violence in nursing is often an under-discussed topic. "An Ontario survey found that in a year, 68% of front-line health workers had been physically assaulted, 86% had faced verbal violence, and 42% had been sexually assaulted or harassed." Many employers will provide you with training on watching for aggressive behaviour how to de-escalate situations. Some even provide training on how to get out of various holds if the patient decides to grab or hit you. This, at the very least, is a step in the right direction. However, the feeling I get from these types of courses is that the safety of the patient is *more important* than the nurses.

We are taught to allow someone to hit us on the softest part of our forearms so they don't hurt themselves, yet we're not trained on making sure *we* don't get hurt. Workplace violence is estimated to affect 58% of nurses in Canada and the United States. For nurses, experiencing some form of violence can be an everyday occurrence depending on where you work. With that in mind, here are ways of coping with that fact and protecting yourself:

1) Be aware of your surroundings—*always*. The art of being aware of my surroundings is something I have always practiced. To be aware, is to be vigilant. I always take note if there are people around me, especially men. I'm aware of hazards, both physical and potential. Is there someone who's a bit too close to me physically? Do I feel uncomfortable, or is someone's tone of voice making me concerned that they may escalate? Be aware of how you feel when assessing a patient. Is the patient making remarks that make you feel uncomfortable or *creep you out*? Is the patient starting to yell or grab you? Are they throwing objects or making threatening comments? Are they making sexually inappropriate comments or saying racist things disguised as jokes? Be aware of how your body responds to your patient, particularly if your gut is saying something is wrong. You can *always* ask (politely) for the patient to stop making the jokes or remarks. You can also be

protective of your own space and, if the patient is getting too close, make sure you have a route to escape. Never close yourself into a space with someone who makes you nervous. Keep your back to the door and never let someone get in-between you and your exit.

2) Alert others if someone is making you uncomfortable. Talk to the charge nurse, a co-worker, or the doctor if there's been a situation that is bothering you. They may provide some perspective, and it might just be a good idea to vent.

3) Don't wear anything around your neck. No lanyards (*especially* if they are not a breakaway lanyard) or necklaces if you're in a high-risk environment. Lanyards also have a habit of getting in the way during messy situations or sterile fields.

4) Unless it's your work's policy, I refuse to have my last name on my badge. It's a safety issue. I work in the emergency room and deal with too many people who I would rather *not* have access to my last name.

5) If someone has overdosed and brought in the prescription bottles with medications still in them, take the medications away from the bedside.

6) Never turn your back on someone who your gut tells you is dangerous or makes you feel unsafe.

7) Always bring in extra hands if you feel delivering some unwelcome news will set the patient or family off. Having support in the room is never a bad thing.

8) Use security if you need them and even better—befriend them! There is no point to having access to security if you don't utilize their services when needed.

9) If someone looks like they're about to yell or get upset, apologize and thank them for being so understanding. This will usually catch people off guard and make them rethink yelling. Most people want to be perceived as the *good person* and will often say it's not a problem. This trick is genius and a game changer in my practice.

6 | VIOLENCE AND SAFETY

10) You are not getting paid to be hit, kicked, spat on, yelled out, cussed out, sexually harassed or otherwise abused. If this is happening, email your manager/boss and *start documenting*. Document in the patient's chart and warn other nurses. Our corporation has a behaviour safety risk tool that allows us to flag abusive behaviors. Also, consider documenting in a journal at home. Don't use patient names, but initials or the individual's age and sex is fine. Describe the situation, the behaviors, what you did about it, and who you notified. You never know when someone will ask for details or if you will need evidence to support your concerns. Trust me on this one.

11) If you are hit or hurt, go to the ER and get checked out. In Canada, we have the Workplace Safety and Insurance Board (WSIB). If you have documentation that you were hurt at work, and if you ever have long-standing issues linked to that injury, you can be compensated while you recover. *We are not paid to get hurt!* Do what you need to do to document the incident and make sure you're covered in the long-term.

12) Getting therapy is key. I believe that everyone who routinely witnesses or is exposed to violence should have access to someone they trust with mental health training. All too often, we become numb to the level of violence we see every day, and it becomes the norm. It should *never* be the norm to deal with what we deal with and see every day. Ask yourself—if someone did this to the police or even a McDonald's employee, what would happen? The answer? The behavior would not be tolerated, and the police would be called. This should also be the case in nursing.

People will react differently to the multitude of things nurses see in a career. Be self-aware and vigilant in monitoring changes in your thoughts and feelings. Talk to coworkers. Empower a colleague to alert you when you aren't acting like yourself. Someone who works with you, and sees you on a regular basis, will be able to tell you if something changes. Are you quicker to judgement? Do you become angry or seem irritated more frequently? Observations like this will tell you that you're not yourself. It may be time to take a step back, reach out for help, and request some much-needed time off.

CASE STUDY

I was working in recovery after experiencing major burnout with the emergency room. I felt it was a safer place. People were happier, thankful, grateful and, above all, were *nice to the nurses*! It was a haven at a time when I needed to take a step back from the ER.

We were getting a patient who would be staying in the recovery unit overnight, as there were no beds in the hospital. We could hear this gentleman yelling from down the hall before he even made it into recovery, which is a closed unit. He was elderly with an underlying history of dementia and had a recent surgery with anesthesia.

He was clearly confused—yelling repeatedly and speaking in another language. There was a group of us trying to get him settled for nightshift. I had to lean over the right side of the bed to put on the oxygen monitor and, before I knew it, the man was swinging his left hand, almost hitting me in the face. I stumbled back, confused as I hadn't seen it coming. Immediately, I was triggered. The violence that I was so used to in the ER had followed me down to the recovery room. What made me the angriest was that I had let my guard down and almost gotten hurt. I had to walk away and collect myself. My heart was racing. I was so *mad* at myself for almost getting hurt when, in the ER, I probably would have had my guard up with someone so agitated.

After a few moments, I returned to the nursing station where the patient was directly in front of me. Thankfully, my colleagues had continued to hook the patient up to the monitor despite his continuous yelling and swinging at anyone and everyone. I made sure the patient was okay, and checked that no one had gotten hurt. It was around this time that the patient's son called, asking for an update.

After telling him that his dad had been moved into the recovery room, the son started to apologize. He said that his dad always got confused going to the hospital, and even more so with anesthesia. He said to do whatever was needed to keep his dad calm, and the nursing staff safe. When he was told that his dad took a swing at a nurse, he was extremely apologetic. He expressed how sorry he was and reiterated that this behaviour was not who his father was. He asked if his dad was speaking English, and we told him that he was not. The son took a deep breath and asked us again, to do whatever was needed to keep everyone safe.

He explained that his dad had been a prisoner of war in Poland during World War II at just eight years old.

This revelation hit me square in the chest, and my heart ached. In that moment, all the fear and anger that I had felt, completely dissolved. How could I be upset with this patient and his behaviour? In that moment, I also felt guilty. The patient clearly had no idea where he was, how old he was, or what was going on. It was a lesson in trying to understand the whole picture of the patient and their previous experiences before jumping to conclusions.

The next day, when I returned to work and saw that the patient was to be moved to a bed on the surgical floor, I made a point of warning the next nurse about the patient's behavior. I also told them the reason behind it, and that the patient was confused about where he was. The nurse on the other end of the line was understanding. I asked her to please relay the message to every other nurse who would be taking care of that patient.

With this job, there is always a risk of violence. I think a lot of it is not reported, because of patients like this example. When people are elderly and confused, we don't see their behaviour as intentionally violent, yet here is still a real element of danger. Violence is still violence. We can still be hurt by these patients. Be aware of the stations you are placed in, and know that *anyone* can surprise you. There are no heroics in taking any type of abuse or harassment. Document violent incidents and report them to your charge nurse and manager so that proper precautions can be taken to protect everyone's safety.

Violence is not just another part of the job.

7 | THE IMPORTANCE OF CALM

HAVE YOU ever noticed that when a child is really upset that likely the child's parents are upset as well? This is an example of the child playing off the parents' emotions. I like to refer to this as the "cycle of stress." You can use your influence as an empathetic individual to influence the behavior of the child. The child and their parents will echo your energy. If you are calm, the parents tend to become calmer. The child sees this and becomes calmer as well.

You can use the cycle of stress and worry to your advantage by turning it into a cycle of calm.

- Use slow deliberate speech.
- Move carefully and with purpose.
- Speak softly while reassuring the parents/caregivers that you are there to help.
- With the child, distraction is your biggest ally—be it a sticker, a blown-up glove or an empty, clean 10cc syringe that you pull into two pieces making a popping sound.

Once everyone is calmer, the child's vital signs will change because they are no longer crying and upset. This will lead to a more accurate representation of the child's *actual* vital signs.

The key is *you*, your attitude. If you remain cool and steady and aren't rushing around, the more people will relax around you. If you act like the child isn't very sick, (though they very well may be) everyone tends to relax. Even if a patient's condition is serious, you can harness the energy of the adrenaline and use it to focus in on what needs to be done.

If you've had a situation where you felt the adrenaline free flowing through your veins, it's scary! Your hands shake, you become uncoordinated, your heart pounds and you feel like you can't think straight.

This is all totally *normal* but can be a lot to handle the first few times. The best thing you can do is to just take a minute before you do, or say, anything. Instead, step back and *breathe*. Drop your shoulders away from your ears, take a deep in-breath and hold for a second or two, then slowly exhale. Think about what you need to do next. Ask for help if needed. (You probably will, so reach out early.)

I've made a handful of comments throughout my career of which I am not proud. In the moment, I thought I was just using a bit of the "tough ER nurse" perspective. Looking back, I know I could've done things differently. Though my words and actions were motivated by the intention of helping the patient, those moments have shown me just how burnt out I was at the time. We'll cover burnout in Chapter 9, but just know that it's an ever-evolving state of being that's never far from the surface. Some weeks you seem fine but then you're triggered by something, and find yourself regretting your actions and wondering why you ever became a nurse.

EXERCISE: MEDITATION

Find a quiet spot and sit comfortably—whether on a chair, sitting up in bed or on the floor. Place a pillow underneath your hips if it makes you more uncomfortable. Quiet your mind. If you find that your mind is racing and you're suddenly trying to find a reason to do anything *other* than sit in the quiet, that's okay. In fact, it's normal. If you're not used to meditation or even to having a minute to yourself, it's understandable if your mind races and your body is restless. Try to let the thoughts pass through your head. Let them float by without expectation. Don't get caught up in each one. If you need to stop and write down a to-do list, then do that! Whatever it takes to quiet your mind.

Drop your shoulders away from your ears, unclench your jaw and take a slow deep inhalation through your nose. Hold for three to four seconds and then exhale through your mouth. If you feel like making noise while exhaling—do it!

Breathe in for four seconds, hold for four seconds and let go for four seconds. This is known as triangle breathing. Focus on the count. Try to

7 | THE IMPORTANCE OF CALM

meditate for a few minutes daily. Start slow and be methodical about it before you lengthen your sessions. Be kind and gentle with yourself.

Practicing meditation is a way to steal back time to care for yourself at home or on a work break. Be aware that unpleasant things may make themselves known. Emotions we've pushed the hardest away are usually the first to re-surface: traumas, codes, difficult patients, times we've lost our cool, and moments that we were later ashamed of all tend to come up in this space of intentional pause.

Use a journal to record your feelings. Don't shy away from hurt, pain and/or anguish. The reason you're feeling it now is because you locked it away until you had a moment to reflect, cope and heal. We all have these parts of ourselves. It's what we do moving forward that makes the difference. We can either turn away from our feelings or acknowledge them. The choice is always ours.

Check in with yourself.

- How are you feeling at this moment?
- Take a deep breath. Are you having any pain or uncomfortable sensations?
- Are you sitting up straight? Are your shoulders up by your ears? Drop them down – how does that feel?
- Is your mind racing with a specific concern or topic?

Time for a brain dump. Write down any concerns as they pop up.

_____
_____
_____
_____
_____
_____
_____
_____

EXERCISE: SQUARE BOX BREATHING

Square box breathing is used by Navy Seals and police in times of stress or conflict. It's a simple technique that takes no time and will help you to become mindful of your breathing.

If I'm having a particularly stressful day or moment, I use this exercise to refocus myself.

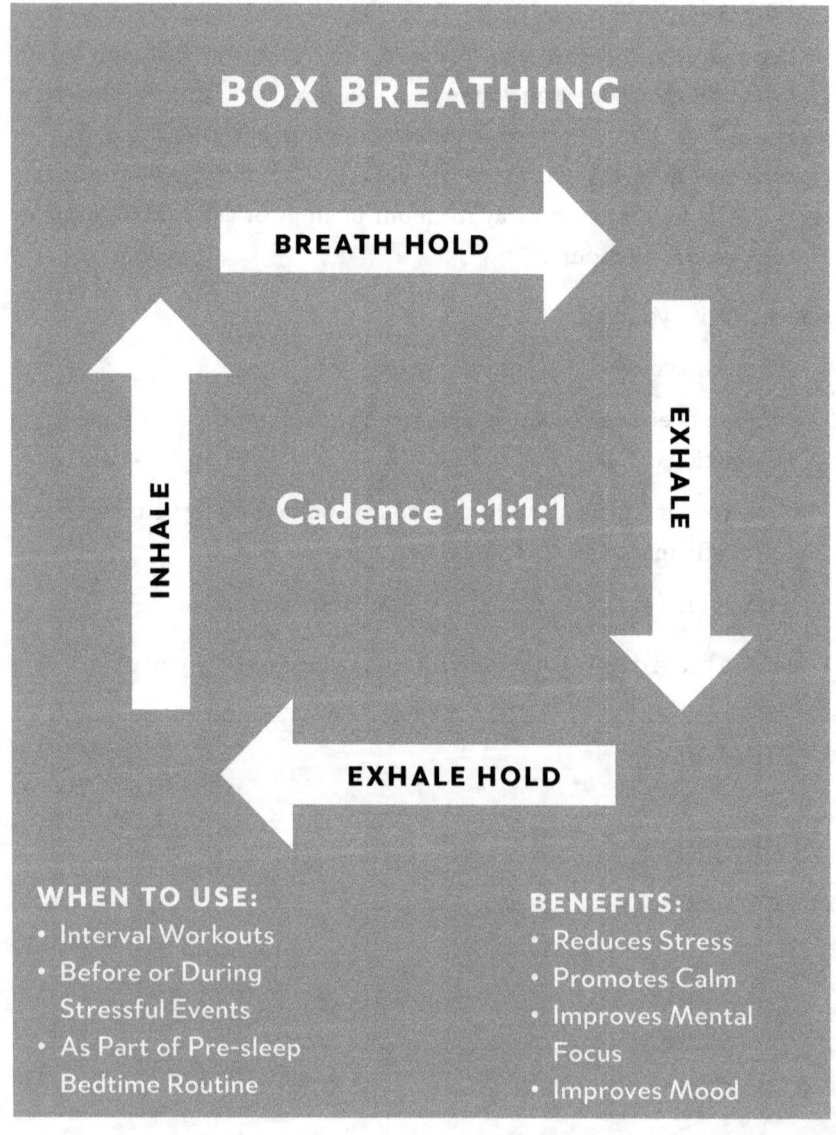

7 | THE IMPORTANCE OF CALM

Sometimes I'm able to hold the bottom count for four. Sometimes it's extraordinarily hard to do that. In that instance, I turn the box into a triangle—inhaling for four, holding for four and exhaling for four before taking an immediate inhale and repeating the process.

Both square box breathing and triangle breathing can be used anywhere for any amount of time, especially if you just need to pause and take a moment to yourself. Find what works best for you and add that to your resilience tool kit.

If you have *more* than a few moments and you want to level this up, you can sit in a quiet space and do a "tightening" exercise. Start with tightening your feet slowly moving that tension up your calves and then thighs, clenching your hips and glutes, abdomen and chest. Feel the constriction in your shoulders and neck. You may find you're curling tightly into yourself. Hold that stress pose for five to ten seconds and then, very consciously, let go of everything in the reverse, shaking it out afterwards.

I understand that within a twelve-hour shift it often feels like you haven't even one second to breathe. I often use the square box breathing while I am charting. Focusing on my breathing in a moment that I am already paused will slow my heart rate and helps to decrease my stress at that moment. Taking a few moments for myself calms my mind so I can focus on whatever comes next.

The key is to figure out what helps *you* to feel better in the few moments that you have in a day. Perhaps when you finally get to take a bathroom break, you can take a minute to pee and box breathe. If I know that a trauma is coming in, I will take a moment to picture what I need to do and what I anticipate happening as people get organized. I prepare the paperwork and box breathe while I do it. It slows my heart and helps me focus.

If all you do now is become aware of those opportunities where you can take a minute to do a box breathing exercise—that's a fantastic start! I know that you're busy. You're run off your feet. You barely get a bathroom break, let alone a chance to eat. I get it. No one has time for lengthy practices that take you off the floor. You don't have the ability to shift your entire focus from the job. But if you dedicate the moments you can—even for just thirty seconds—to bring awareness to your breathing, you will be better prepared to identify what is going on in your body.

"Do what you can when you can," that's the ER motto. Think of how many times you quickly check your phone. Those check-ins would probably add up to five to ten minutes in a 12-hour shift. Try focusing on your breathing instead of scrolling.

Take a minute now to try square box breathing.

8 | MEDICAL WITH A SPRINKLE OF MAGICAL

I'VE EXPERIENCED many *ah-ha* moments in my career. These occurrences have taught me—with flashes of insight—that the world is *not* as black and white as it seems. The events may seem ordinary to someone else, but to *me* they were *extra*ordinary and changed my whole perspective on a situation. Take, for example, the first time I heard a baby cry after being born.

Suddenly, and overwhelmingly, there was a feeling of magic in the air. A new life had been brought into the world and not only was I there, I witnessed this birth happen – the *whole thing*. From the first peek of the baby's hair, thinking *aww that's it,* to feeling *astonishment* as the baby was pushed out. I realized (incredibly) just how *large* that baby's head was. It was then that it hit me. It was *insane* that a baby came *out* of her like that! In my student-nurse daze, I watched the cord being cut and the baby being placed on mom's chest. I saw the moment of understanding pass between mom and dad, that their whole life had changed in an instant. (Now having had two children of my own, I know that their lives truly changed about 8 1/2 months prior to the birth when they found out they were pregnant, but I was too young to think about that at the time.)

After that, that I started to look for the magical parts of nursing. Granted they are few and far between, but when you feel it, you feel it deep. Catching someone on the tipping point of death—and then pulling them back from the brink. Following my gut about a concern—and then being right. "Shocking" someone, who is technically dead, and bringing them back to life. Nursing truly can be magical.

Getting to support a patient or their family as they withdraw care can also be magical. Palliative care is a personal love of mine, and I received a certificate in palliative care before graduating nursing. Being able to provide support, in life and in death, is what we are here to do. It's an honor. It's also terribly traumatic at times...but we'll get to that.

Nursing is many things. In one moment, you're an angel to a patient—holding their hand and sharing in their misery. In the next, you're being called names (none of them angel) by another patient who you've refused to give narcotics. So, you become hardened to the stresses and the daily grind and misery of your unit until there is a moment that shocks you into remembering why you do this in the first place. It's at that point, when you open your heart to release your deeply hidden empathy and compassion, that magical things can happen. And they do happen. Far more often than we realize. It's up to us to be present enough to witness it.

CASE STUDY

It was the height of the pandemic. Visits to our emergency room had declined significantly, but the acuity had gone up as people were putting off coming into the hospital unless they were extremely ill. This was the case for the patient who had rung the call bell and I was the only one available to answer it. The patient was in isolation as according to the COVID screening she had symptoms that could be linked to COVID. I gowned-up, privately wondering if this was the person who was going to expose me to COVID and if I would get ill, or worse—make my family sick. In addition to my gown, my hair was covered in a bright scrub cap with a universe pattern and I wore safety goggles over my glasses and a plastic shield over my face, I was sweating before I even entered the room. Pull back the curtain revealed the silhouette of a frail elderly body, curled up into a fetal position. I could see that their respiration rate was already elevated and their color was green/pale. They looked like they were struggling to breathe. I tried to get vitals but was unable to get a blood pressure. Their pulse was in the forties and their oxygen level was in the eighties. I'm assessing, but I already know this is anything but a good situation for the patient. The ER doctor pops his head in the door.
"Hey Jenn, are you in there?" he asks.

"Yes. What's the plan with this patient? Their respiration rate is up, SpO2 is down, and I can't for the life of me get a blood pressure." My voice nearly wavers and I'm worried that other patients have overheard my question.

8 | MEDICAL WITH A SPRINKLE OF MAGICAL

"It says here that they are from a long-term care home and came in for shortness of breath," he informs me blankly, looking at the chart. "Do you need something for the breathing?" He looks at me, his head cocking to the side.

"Actually...if they are from a long-term care home, are there advanced directives? I think the patient is trying to pass," I say bluntly.

"It looks like they've been in palliative care for a few days, then their breathing changed so the nursing staff were concerned and sent them in."

Ugh. I inwardly curse. It's obvious that the patient is in the last stages of dying and clearly the staff were either not comfortable with them being there or were thinking something else (like COVID) was going on. The patient's breathing is fast, laboured, and they're not responding to voice or touch. Their pulse is starting to slow down and the longer I stand there, the clearer it is that they're no more than thirty minutes away from dying. I ask my doctor for some sedation or pain medication. He says he will have someone draw it up for me as we were trying to limit the number of times staff entered different isolation rooms in the ER.

I think about what else could be done, thankfully reminding myself that my section of the department was empty, giving me the time to sit with the patient. I poke my head out of the room to ask my charge nurse if anyone has contacted the family and if they had been notified of the patient's deteriorating condition.

"Not yet," she replies.

"Can we give them a call? It's 5 am and I doubt that the long-term care home has called them."

"Sounds good," my charge nurse nods. "We'll try and track them down and update them. How long do you think we have?"

"Not long. Get them in here as soon as possible if they would like to say their goodbyes," I quietly say.

I return to the room and pull up a chair by the patient. I lower the rail of the stretcher and pulled the chair even closer. I hold the patient's hand, though my gloves prevent me from feeling their skin. Looking again, I notice their emaciated frame tenting the thin white sheet. I see their eyes, open but not focusing. Their breathing has begun to slow, having longer pauses in between shallow breaths. Who was this tiny shadow of a person? What had their life been like? What were their dreams and fears?

I didn't know so I began to fill in the gaps.

I imagined they were my grandparent, close to death with my family not having enough time to get there for their last moments. I pictured the patient with a loving family, having led a full life with many moments of joy throughout. I saw them in their prime, raising children in the same way I was now and wondered how that comparison could stand. Maybe we weren't so different after all? Just one of us a little more ahead of the other.

Time passed. I noted again that the patient's breathing was continuing to slow with pauses becoming longer, and their pulse slowing. I told them it was okay to go, that I was there so that they weren't alone. It's a personal mantra that no one dies alone in my ER. Not if I could help it.

I can only imagine the fear and other thoughts that go through someone's mind as they die. Do they know what's happening, or are they blissfully unaware? Thankfully this patient didn't seem to be in pain as I was still waiting for pain and sedation medication from my colleagues. I just sat there, holding their hand and rubbing the back of it. It got to the point where the patient was on the cusp of death. I brushed their hair back and told them it was okay.

I've witnessed a lot of death in my years but had never been the only one present to hold their hand as someone died. I watched the patient breathe their last breath. I watched the life drain from their eyes. I watched as their face relaxed and their head fell to the side. It was unsettling, but it was *peaceful*.

My eyes started to burn, letting me know that tears were on their way. It was all I could do to take off my isolation gear in proper order before the tears started to fall. I needed a minute to collect myself and got halfway down the hallway to the break room when I realized that I forgot to let the soul out.

I believe that when someone dies, their soul is released and I like to help direct it to the outdoors as we never have windows in the ER that we can open. I returned to the room, opened the door a crack and said out loud: "I'm sorry, but sadly you have died. This was your time. If your soul would like to follow me, I'm going to take it outside."

8 | MEDICAL WITH A SPRINKLE OF MAGICAL

I make a "follow me" motion with my hands at the door and walk towards the exit. My charge nurse is standing there, and I know she's heard me but thankfully she says nothing. I think most of the nurses I've worked with have figured out my quirks. I buzz myself through the two sliding doors to go outside and stand in the ambulance bay. I feel a rush of cool air pass behind me and am reminded that it's a drizzly, cloudy, dark early morning.

I look to my left and see brooding storm clouds with faint rumblings of thunder in the distance. I turn to my right and notice, what seems to be, a hole in the clouds. This strikes me as odd, as the entire sky was one giant angry storm cloud waiting to pelt us with rain. Then I saw it. The most beautiful and well-defined rainbow I'd ever seen, breaking through the clouds. It was then that I fully lost it. I cried, looking up at the rainbow and knew it was my patient. I rushed inside to tell the others about the gorgeous rainbow, inviting them back outside to enjoy a happy moment but it was already gone. I realize then that the rainbow was for me, and me alone. I like to think of it as a thank you from the patient. I smile, my sadness still there but less profound. The patient was at peace and I'd had a role in helping them find that.

It was a win, and I took it.

9 | HOW TO PROTECT YOUR ENERGY

THERE HAVE BEEN so many times in nursing where I was pushed to do more than I felt comfortable doing—multiple instances where I felt I was stretched thin and pushed to the point of breaking. For some reason though, I treated being overworked as a point of pride. I thought that being tired and still accepting more shifts was me *showing up*, like some kind of superhero. I acted like exhaustion was something I could just push past, completely ignoring my intuition.

I was a new grad, young and eager to prove my worth. I would say yes to things because —

a) I was unable to say no, and
b) I didn't even realize I *could* say no.

It was never talked about—the fact that work will call and call, asking more of you than you ever thought possible. You may want to say no, but end up feeling guilty because you know what it's like to be short-staffed. The "be a hero" complex kicks in. All for just showing up! And, let's face it, overtime pay is nothing to sneeze at either. I didn't realize I was setting a precedent for myself. By never saying no, by talking myself out of saying no, I thought I was strong! I thought, *I'm not tired, it's no big deal* and besides what was I going to do today *anyways*?

At the time I also didn't realize how awful the culture was at my hospital. The hospital was so small that there was only one registered nurse for the emergency department. That's right – one. No other support staff, so most of the time it was just me receiving the patient, triaging them, doing their orders, giving the medications and then discharging them home.

Now, to be fair, the town was under 5,000 people. Generally, we would see less than ten patients in a shift (sometimes none in a nightshift). It meant there was time to tend all the patients and I wasn't run off my feet but if something major happened, it was just me in the department unless I called the floor and asked for help. Again, the floor only had one registered nurse and two registered practical nurses, so the availability of help was limited. Sometimes we would call in the next shift early (another way to get overworked, stretching a twelve-hour shift into a fifteen- or sixteen-hour shift).

I started to realize I couldn't "do it all" after routinely accepting a shift that had me "double backing" —you work a night shift, get off the next morning and then return for a day shift. Double backs are so named because you are short-changing yourself sleep, and time to get your body back into dayshift mode after working nights. It's a young person's game. I found that the more double backs I did, the more tired, cranky, and generally foul mood I would be in for most of that dayshift. In the end, they weren't worth the effort as my energy and well-being were worth more than what I would be paid for that shift.

The biggest question for me, when it comes to my energy, is asking what I'm sacrificing by doing overtime. Is it worth more than what I would be doing at home? Am I having to reschedule appointments or make changes to plans to go into work? Now, if I have something booked, I answer no. I realized that I was tired of rebooking appointments made months prior. I even started to make appointments so that it was roughly one appointment a day that I was off. That way I was *forced* to say no to the shift. I noticed that I felt better when I wasn't worked to death and picking up every shift possible and I wasn't constantly on alert for a call to come in.

I also realized that when I was at work and having a rough day, that I would look ahead to my days off and make plans. I would have to amp myself up to feel as if I was strong enough to say no if work called. It was a constant battle between feeling like you had to answer the phone in order to be "a good employee" but then dreading going in. I would start to preplan excuses as to why I couldn't come in. Things like "I have an appointment, I've made plans." It got to the point where I would pre-plan excuses as to why I couldn't come in because my phone was usually ringing off the hook for shift pickups. The guilt felt never ending as the push and pull between what I thought was expected and what I could emotionally do felt at odds.

To be honest, it took me over a decade to be able to just say no to a shift without automatically giving an excuse. I just got so tired of explaining myself, and I'm sure the schedulers got tired of hearing the excuses. So, I just started saying no and the result left me feeling empowered about putting my mental health first!

As nurses we're taught to always think of others, but after years of putting everyone else's needs and expectations ahead of my own finally caught up with me. I started to resent work. I started to dread coming in, wondering how badly I would be pushed to the limit. I counted down the 12 hours of shift, thinking about how I would have to go straight to bed and then do it all over again. Don't get me wrong. I still prefer twelve-hour shifts over eight-hour shifts, where it feels like there isn't enough time in the week to get all the things done that I want to.

FINDING RESILIENCE

There are many ways to start protecting your energy and realize when you need to take a step back. Making small changes can increase resilience and thus, make you less likely to experience burnout. Resilience is defined as "the ability to 'rebound' from adversity when one's ability to function has been to some degree impaired." In other words, resilience is a measurement of someone's ability to take daily emotional wear and tear based on how well they are taking care of themselves. It gives us a concrete idea that we *do* need to be mindful of how much we're taking on and how we are coping.

Consider the following behaviours. Do any apply to you? If so, burnout may be simmering closer to the surface than you realized.

1. You're short with everyone, even your favorite co-workers.

2. *Everything* is an effort. Answering the call bell immediately brings a "what now?" kind of reaction.

3. You're sleeping less, more fitfully, not able to fall asleep, or not able to stay asleep.

4. You're dreading going into work.

5. Pulling up to park, or walking up in the door of your workplace causes physical reactions: your chest tightens, you get sweaty and your breathing quickens. You're approaching a panic attack.

6. You're starting to use unhealthy coping mechanisms like food, alcohol, drugs, sex, gambling, and other high-risk behaviours.

7. You, and those around you, notice you're not acting like yourself. Some may ask if you're okay. You know something is wrong, but you're not willing to deal with it.

9 | HOW TO PROTECT YOUR ENERGY

EXERCISE: BURNOUT ALERT

Of the behaviours listed, what resonates with you in your current situation?

_____
_____
_____
_____

What statement felt the truest for you?

_____
_____
_____
_____

What's your current coping mechanism?

_____
_____
_____
_____

Is it working? And does it offer long-term benefits?

_____
_____
_____
_____

Do you have a support network?

_____
_____
_____
_____

Why or why not?

_____
_____
_____
_____

How could you develop a support network or strengthen the one you currently have?

_____
_____
_____
_____

What's one easy change that would help to make your home life better?

_____
_____
_____
_____

What have you been meaning to do but haven't found the time or energy?

_____
_____
_____
_____

Are you ready to start a plan to do something that you really enjoy?

_____
_____
_____
_____

10 | INTUITION STORY TIME

HERE'S A QUICK and fun story about intuition. Sometimes intuition will hit you at the oddest times. One of the ER's I worked in had a long hallway that led towards an exit. Sometimes there were stretchers filled with people in this hallway when our bed capacity was full. This hallway was also the spot we regularly let people sober up before heading home. It was early in the morning, and we had a patient who was waiting to do just that. She looked much older than her stated age, her clothes were stiff with the dirt and grime of months (if not years) of not being washed. The woman looked to be homeless and acted every bit the part, calling me over with an expletive. Generally, calling me a bitch is *not* the way to get a response but it was the middle of the night and the 2 am giggles were starting to pop up.

She asked me to come over again, but dropped the bitch from her request. I finished the bit of charting I was working on and walked towards her. The hallway was dimly lit to try and allow stretcher patients some semblance of sleep, which still never happened. The trauma bays were right across from this hallway and traumas always came in just as you'd settle people in for the night. I kept an arm's length away as I asked what she needed.

"I need a drink," she slurred, making a move as if she wanted to tip over the side of the bed. Thankfully the side rails were elevated and prevented her from falling face first onto the floor.

"I can get you some water. Do you want ice?" I asked, tilting my head for that extra perceived effect of *really*?!

"No ice……please," she managed.

I retrieved the water and when I returned to give it to her, she again reached out her arm and almost fell off the stretcher. She also exposed a lower part of her leg covered in ropey scars that looked a bit like scar tissue from burns – but not quite.

"What did you do, put your foot through a plate glass window?" I asked, the words tumbling out of my mouth before I even realized what I was saying.

"How did you know?" her look betraying shock at my guess.

"I'm psychic," I winked and walked away. I chuckled at myself for being glib, but inside I wondered where that information had come from. It just popped into my head and I'd casually blurted it out. It was one of the first instances that I said something to someone where I wasn't thinking at all of what I was saying.

I realized I was picking up on more of someone's story than I thought I was.

11 | CAREGIVER FATIGUE AND MORAL DISTRESS

YOU have a new demon; one who always lurks in the background and will likely follow you around for the rest of your career. Left unchecked, this demon could very easily cost you your nursing career. Burnout and caregiver fatigue are roller coasters in nursing. One day you are feeling okay, dealing with the daily stresses of life and nursing and then the next you're dealt a mentally challenging situation that can leave lasting scars. These are experiences we all eventually end up having, that follow and haunt us. They become the stories that no one wants to hear but are pressing to be told. The ones that keep you up at night. Those who work as police, in firefighting, EMS and nursing all know this demon. The fact that I am wondering if I should share mine lets you know that we all struggle. But we can't hold them in, carrying them alone, forever.

Burnout has been defined as feelings of hopelessness and difficulties in dealing with work and is known to make up of feelings of emotional exhaustion, depersonalization and reduced personal accomplishment. It is modifiable if improvements occur in the working conditions of nursing staff. Burnout can be associated with complex workload and/or a non-supportive work environment.

I once had a patient ask me, what was the story that kept me up at night? I had only just met this woman—it was almost the first thing out of her mouth. I asked if she really wanted to know, and when she said yes, I told her a very condensed version of a story that still shakes me to my core. Afterward, I thought it was an interesting idea to open a discussion with my colleagues about their dark stories but sometimes this isn't a good idea as everyone is in various stages of coping with their traumas. You need to know your audience before you start asking about their worst nursing experiences. I still hesitate before sharing my dark story. There is power in sharing our lived experiences but also a lot of pain and, truly, you never know who is going to be triggered.

If you do not want to read my story, I invite you to skip forward to the next chapter. There is no test, quiz or follow up questions about it. If you proceed forward and find after that it triggers you, please reach out for help. Find your local therapist or reach out to an employee assistance program that may be offered by your employer. Know that you are not alone in the pain that you carry and that we're all here for each other. It's been many years since my experience and even thinking about it makes me tremble. I can feel the anxiety rising, and my heart starting to race and my hands shake. I'm already on the verge of tears. The pain never goes away. We *all* struggle with something. Know this.

THIS IS MY DARK STORY
Trigger Warning – Pediatric Code

It was an unusually warm night and very early in the morning. It was a shift I wasn't even supposed to be there for, but I'd picked it up as overtime. I planned to go home at 6 am because I hadn't had a break, and the charge had agreed to let me leave early.

It was at 5:55 am when the patch phone rang. A very young child with vital signs absent was on their way in with EMS.

After getting the patch and letting out a silent prayer that things would be okay, I asked my charge nurse if she wanted me to stay because I was the one with the most pediatric experience. My heart sank at her affirmative response. I knew in my gut that this experience was going to stay with me for a lifetime.

We quickly moved patients out of the resuscitation area to make way for the child coming in. Housekeeping and nurses bustled around trying to get the area cleaned and switched over to child-sized equipment. The paediatric code cart was brought out and placed beside the head of the bed. The Braslow tape was affixed to the stretcher to be able to quickly assess the size of the child and then have the corresponding color drawer on the paediatric code cart opened. The dark red plastic lock with its squared white painted on numbers waited for me. I snapped it off and dust came up in that moment, making me even more aware that we hadn't had a paediatric code in a very long time.

11 | CAREGIVER FATIGUE AND MORAL DISTRESS

The monitor was turned on and changed to paediatric settings. The smallest of defibrillator pads we had were hooked up to the defibrillator monitor. Oxygen was checked and a child sized non-rebreather mask attached. Suction was checked and turned on; a smaller size suction catheter attached to the end. The smallest blood pressure cuff we had attached to the monitor was switched on and ready to go. Child-sized intubation equipment appeared half the size of what we normally would use. For every piece of equipment that we changed over, the reality of what was about to happen settled in. The noise volume within the department turned down, a shift in demeanor by the staff as they anticipated the arrival of the tiny patient.

As we waited for EMS to arrive, several nurses, a respiratory therapist as well as the physician surrounded the empty stretcher looking at the equipment. We silently prayed for a miracle, hoping hoped that we had heard the EMS report incorrectly.

It was my first paediatric code, something I could never really prepare for.

EMS finally arrived and the small, limp, blue, lifeless body was placed on the stretcher gently by the paramedics. I started chest compressions. At the time I thought about how little effort it took to squeeze the tiny chest in between my fingers and thumbs.

Wearing nothing more than a wet diaper, I knew that the baby wasn't coming back but I pushed the thought aside, hoping for that miracle. The report from EMS was that the family had checked on the child in the middle of the night and found her in the crib with a blanket, covered in vomit. They called 911. They didn't know how long she'd been without a pulse. If there is anything that can make this type of story even more traumatic, it was the fact that my daughter was the same age at the time this happened.

When EMS arrived, the child already had an intraosseous (IO) line in place to her shin, but it looked like it was no longer working as the cold muscles under the IO started to swell. A second IO was placed in the humeral head, and we were able to start running fluids and push epinephrine.

We worked for what seemed like forever on this tiny body. Round after round of epinephrine and chest compressions. It didn't take long to intubate, and it seemed there was a large amount of vomit in the lungs.

For those of you who routinely work a code with the same people, you know that when you get into that group, you can run codes easily and efficiently. You end up talking about things during the code situation that sometimes have nothing to do with the lifesaving procedures at hand. You work so well together as a group that you're reading each other's minds as to what is to happen next. It's routine. It's predictable. You yell for what you need. You yell to update who's charting. It's usually a very loud, boisterous act.

In this code you could hear a pin drop. No one said a word unless it was needed to be said.

We did everything we possibly could for an hour, but the outcome, sadly, was not a happy one. With the calling of time of death, we all were finally able to take a step back and take a good look at the child. There were bruises where bruises shouldn't be. The report that we got from EMS and what we were looking at didn't match up. A *non-accidental* death was what popped into my head.

The memory of this child haunts me still. The trauma of that night never too far away from the surface of my soul. The sound of the mother screaming afterwards will never leave my memory. I'll always be able to hear her.

All I could think about was getting home and regardless of what time it was, waking up my daughter to sit with her, rock her and tell her I loved her—potentially never letting her out of my arms if I could help it.

After forty-eight hours, I was smart enough to reach out to my employee assistance program for help. My contact told me what types of behaviours to watch out for in relation to post traumatic stress disorder (PTSD) and above all, she comforted me. It was the first time that I was the one being comforted and not the other way around. It was nice, but a little unsettling, causing me to feel that I had lost the sense of "control" over my situation. I was just along for the ride. Things settled and I believed that I was over it. I pushed the memories to the far corners of my mind and told myself I had healed.

The trauma of this code and the pain left in its wake, wrecked me for a long time. It wasn't until years later that I started therapy for a completely unrelated issue, that I even realized it still bothered me. My therapist asked me very gingerly in the beginning stages of therapy if I'd had any trauma in my life.

I was quick to say, "God no, I've been so lucky..." and then I stopped. That child popped into my head. "There was a thing at work a few years ago – but I'm sure it's nothing," I said, waving it off.

Sure enough, it was still something.

Talking about that child and the code to my therapist, was probably the first time I'd said anything about it out loud to another person. I always worried about putting my sad story into the mind of someone else. I didn't want to burden anyone else with the knowledge of such an event. As I finally talked about that code, I cried. I cried *a lot*. I cried for a patient I thought I'd failed.

My therapist said to tell that child all the things that I wanted to say but hadn't through the years.

I said I was sorry. *So sorry*.

I said I was sorry I couldn't protect them and that I couldn't bring them back.

My therapist then suggested that I let the child go. I thought, *okay, but how*? My therapist said to think of something that you can wrap them in. My own kids had Tula blankets—the softest blankets I've ever felt. So, I imagined wrapping that little body, full of life, in the blanket with the utmost of care, taking time to brush the hair off her face and tuck it behind an imaginary ear. I envisioned happiness for the child. Seeing the sweet chubby little body clean and without bruises. I kept saying I was sorry, that I couldn't have done more. I envisioned the child going up into a white light, being safe, and well taken care of.

It helped. The child wasn't as close to the forefront of my daily thoughts. The trauma of that day and the memory of the child is always going to be with me. It was a memory that used to cause so much pain. Now, I envision that little angel being with me if I bring up those memories, but the memory is further back behind me and to the left.

As I write this, tears are streaming down my face. It's the part of nursing that nobody talks about. The pain and trauma and anguish that we carry. There wasn't a class about how to care for that part of ourselves.

Talking about the experience has lessened the pain, removing the weight of it off my chest and freeing me of a burden I've carried for too long.

Having people understand where my head is at makes it easier. Trusting someone with that story makes it easier. Telling dark stories is difficult. Nobody (myself included) wants to be vulnerable, but we need to start sharing as a way to let each other know that none of us are alone. We have similar experiences, including their painful after-effects. There is no point in being strong when it comes to this. We need to talk with each other, and we need to truly listen.

TRAUMA BONDING

I tell my coworkers, EMS, police, and fire that we're all on the same team. Our team *gets it* when we talk about the struggles of dealing with the public, how frustrating it can sometimes be and how we witness things on the regular that *no one* should have to witness. *I* refer to it as trauma bonding. With repeated exposures to traumatic events and circumstances, we develop better understanding of where each other is coming from. We understand dark humor and the early signs of burnout and fatigue. We're very aware when someone's comments or humor get a bit too dark or worrisome.

To be honest we see our co-workers just as much (if not more) than our actual family members, so we know when something's up. To be a person who is comfortable enough with their own trauma, to be able to support someone else who may be struggling, is a gift. Working in nursing can be more than overwhelming at times, and even more so since Covid-19.

Too often we run on autopilot: going to work, coming home and sleeping just enough before going back to work once more. Days off are spent catching up on mundane household chores trying to keep your household afloat. Know that sometimes all it takes is a kind word asking if you're okay to make you sit back and ask yourself the same question. *So, ask the question!*

11 | CAREGIVER FATIGUE AND MORAL DISTRESS

I challenge you to ask 1-2 people you work with, who you think may be struggling, if they're okay. They may brush you off and try to continue with their day. *Don't let them.* Get them to *stop* and *look* at you. Look into their eyes and truly ask if they're okay. A few things could happen—

a) They continue to say that they're okay.

b) They are taken by surprise but want to talk about it.

c) They think about it and may *not want to* talk about it.

d) They may break down. Be prepared, as it may be the most likely option to happen. All you need to do is be there. Listen with an open mind.

All these reactions can also happen with the same person if you were to ask them on different days and in different situations. Unless it's in a situation where someone is clearly struggling at work, I suggest the conversation be done in private. Ask someone to come over for a drink and a vent session or going out to grab a bite to eat are great ways to get people talking.

I keep harping on this idea that we need to support each other because *we do*. No other person can understand how truly hard it is to work in nursing than those who work alongside you. No one better understands the stresses you face every day than your co-workers.

"Working together in this fight leads to a great camaraderie between team members, and these bonds between team members' matter."

Support each other.

JOURNAL PROMPTS

What's your trauma?
___
___
___
___

Have you seen someone about it? Talked to friends or family about it?
___
___
___
___

Why or why not?
___
___
___
___

12 | EXERCISES FOR RESILIENCE

AS I TALK about the heavy things, I might as well give you some tips on how to cope with the situations you'll be faced with. We all know that to nurse is to experience someone else's misery, and then smile for the next patient as if nothing has happened. It's these types of situations where you must put your feelings on pause where the risk for long-term emotional damage increases.

DEBRIEFING

Debriefing is not counselling. It's a "structured voluntary discussion aimed at putting an abnormal event into perspective. It offers workers clarity about the critical incident they have experienced and assists them to establish a process for recovery."

In a perfect world, debriefing would happen immediately after the event to give everyone who participated a chance to decompress. It's also a way to help the team build on their experiences and grow from them. In a debrief, everyone is asked to present their version of what happened—what went right, what went wrong and how it could be improved for next time. This gives a 360 view of an event and lets everyone know they are not alone in their feelings about what transpired. It's a no-judgement zone to support one another.

Usually, a debrief is hosted at the end of the shift and everyone who was involved in the incident participates. It's never mandatory, but rather voluntary. It's difficult after a grueling shift. Normally you just want to get home and go to bed, but if your workplace is offering a debrief, I *highly* suggest you attend for your mental health and learning. Hearing from your co-workers that nothing more could've been done, or knowing (for a fact) that nothing was missed will take a worry off your mind. You may need to hear that there wasn't anything more you personally could have done, especially for new nurses who might not have experienced a traumatic event. A debrief provides learning moments within the supportive environment of your managers and co-workers.

Trained debrief staff can help workers to explore and understand a range of issues, including:

- the sequence of events
- the causes and consequences
- each person's experience
- any memories triggered by the incident
- normal psychological reactions to critical incidents
- methods to manage emotional responses resulting from a critical incident

GRATITUDE JOURNAL

A gratitude journal can be a great way to (quickly) practice self-care. It only takes a minute to write down something that you're grateful or thankful for. One line - that's it. It seems simple and too good to be true—I know. All it requires is a journal that you put somewhere in view as you get ready for the day: the kitchen counter, your bedside table, or in your bathroom. Then, writing a quick one liner about what you're grateful for is all it takes. It may be about family, your job, having a warm bed—it all counts. Some days it may take a minute to identify your gratitude thought, but it gets easier with time. Your entries will vary day-to-day, and you may be surprised what comes to mind, flowing freely to the page.

MEDITATION

We've all heard about the benefits of meditation. There are many studies that show the benefits of this practice. In theory, I'm all for meditation. As a mother of a five and seven-year-old, I find that carving out time for myself is damn near impossible, let alone it being quiet and reflective enough for meditation. However, should you find yourself in a moment where you have a few quiet (yes, I said the Q-word) minutes, try the following steps to find focus and calm your thoughts.

12 | EXERCISES FOR RESILIENCE

- Sit comfortably with your back straight.
- Breath in through your nose and out through your mouth.
- Breathe easily as you notice how you're feeling.
- Try to slow your breathing to also slow down your heart rate. Observe the effect.
- Feel your heart beat, knowing that it's within your control to slow your racing heart.
- Let your breath come in and out as it wants. All you're trying to do in the moment is slow your heart rate.
- You will be bombarded with thoughts. Try to let them pass you by.
- If you become distracted, re-focus on your breathing. Come back to your breath.

If you're new to meditation, try it for just a few minutes at a time. Weekly would be optimal for those of us struggling to find a few minutes of peace.

"The least you can do is give it a try!"

THERAPY

I used to think that therapy was for the weak and for those who had much bigger problems than I perceived I had. Then I actually went and tried a therapy session. It has been (by far) the most beneficial tool for me in building coping mechanisms. There is no judgement in therapy, only an ear that is neutral and willing to help.

I've had two therapists and they've each helped me in their own way. With both, I had an opportunity to express what I had been too scared to say to my co-workers or friends. I didn't want to burden them so I just pushed my feeling away. Not dealing with my struggles in a timely manner did me a huge disservice. In therapy I realized that there was more to what I was feeling, than the issues I was having with those I loved outside of work.

Eventually, if you work with the public, you will be put into a situation where you could benefit from therapy – I'm going to leave it at that.

Do what you're comfortable with, but know everyone can benefit from therapy and if you're paying into benefits and not using them—that's a damn shame.

SLEEP

With shiftwork and the swing back and forth between nights, days, and weekends—are you getting enough sleep?

EXERCISE - SLEEP ASSESSMENT

Are you able to *get to* sleep? _____

Are you able to *stay* asleep? _____

How long do you normally sleep after dayshift? _____

After nightshift if going into another nightshift? _____

After nightshift if it's your last nightshift? _____

Do you have a sleep routine? _____

Describe it: _____
_____

Do you have nightmares? _____

Describe them: Are there themes that repeat?
_____
_____

Do you wake up in a panic or drenched in sweat? How often? _____
_____

Do you take medication to help you go to, or stay asleep? _____

What are they? Do they work? _____
_____

12 | EXERCISES FOR RESILIENCE

Do you have a routine for preparing for night shift?
_____

Describe it: _____

_____

Do you take a lot of double back (switching from nights to days within 24 hrs) shifts? _____

How often do you feel exhausted? _____

_____

Is sleep the best part of your day? _____

_____

Do you dream of work, call bells, or alarms ringing? _____

_____

When I started therapy, I was struggling more than I ever had before. I had just switched to straight nights to accommodate the fact that with COVID, we no longer had daycare and no access to anyone to watch our two children. The plan was for me to work nights, come home and watch the kids until my husband came home. I would nap for as long as I could and go back in for my next shift. As you can imagine this was not sustainable. Thankfully, a local university student association started a volunteer program where frontline staff could have a volunteer assigned to them to help with activities like grocery runs, dog sitting and other much-needed tasks. Even childcare would be available, allowing frontline staff the ability to continue working during the first wave of the COVID pandemic.

This was a blessing to someone with small children and no other access to childcare. I was assigned two of the sweetest people I could've asked for. Bianca was in her last year of nursing school and Srimann was finishing up a teaching degree. These two sweet angels watched my children *for free* while I slept after nightshifts. I still only got four to five hours of sleep because I didn't want to abuse the gift I'd been given. Often, with the decrease in ER visits during the first wave, we were able to go for a rest on our break during nightshift, which also helped but ultimately, my sleep was fractured and "quality sleep" was non-existent.

Knowing that sleep plays a huge factor in our overall wellness is something we like to gloss over as shift workers. Once again there is an, *I can do it all* mentality. We even take pride in the suffering. It's a ridiculous mental framework that needs to change. How can we possibly take care of others when we are barely taking care of ourselves?

EXERCISE

Yes, I know. Who am I to suggest exercise when the thought of breaking a sweat anywhere other than at work isn't likely to happen? (I admit, you'll hear me refer to the couch as my "bestie.") If you are someone who uses exercise to feel better, *I applaud you*! Seriously. I wish this is how I felt about exercise.

There was a point where I started to view exercise (and the endorphins it produces) as a medication for the depression I was clearly in, but refused to acknowledge. I started to run, which helped, considering it my antidepressant. Within the last few months, I have become non-compliant and continue to struggle at getting back to running semi-regularly. If you can ease your way into exercise, I would suggest a focus on increasing strength in your back and core. Back issues are common for most bedside nurses by the middle of our careers.

UNHEALTHY COPING MECHANISMS

It's time to take a quick peek at the things we are using to *decompress* after a long day. These are things that may help in the moment but if left unchecked, can cause even bigger problems.

- Alcohol
- Substance misuse and abuse
- Over/under eating
- Over/under sleeping
- Gambling

- Game addictions
- Phone addiction
- Sex addiction
- Hiding or avoiding family or friends (hermiting)

Usually what helps in the short term, can end up being a much larger problem in the long term.

13 | HABITS AND RITUALS

HAVE YOU EVER met a nurse that *doesn't* have habits relating to the job? I've known nurses who like to come in early and research their patients before report; who go in order of room numbers; who asks a million questions during report; or doesn't ask a question at all.

Everyone starts their careers doing tasks a certain way based on their schooling, their personal background, and their clinical experiences. Some will figure out what works for them while others will seemingly be in a state of chaos their entire career. Being organized can completely change the course of your day and as you get more experience, you will likely find your groove. It's when you're suddenly thrust into a situation that takes you out of your norm that things can fall off the rails. This is a summary of my thought process as I get organized for a day shift—my *shift ritual* if you will.

FOOD

If I don't pack several snacks that can be eaten quickly, on the go or at the very least, kept in my pocket as I work, I'm a goner. Also: Coffee is life.

MUSIC

I have an *ER pump up* playlist on my phone (see Appendix). It's a mix of high energy music and it gets me in the mood for running around like a maniac. I feel empowered as I walk into work and my vibe is: "I've got this. Let's kick some ass." The music lifts my spirits and I *love* a good beat drop. My mood is set for success and I start prepared for another day in the ER.

PENS

I will always have a minimum of two to three pens (click top preferred) on me. If you are missing a pen, I have it and I'm not sorry.

COMPRESSION STOCKINGS

Especially with a dayshift (where I'm running for most of the day) compression stockings are a lifesaver and covered by our benefits. My feet aren't aching at the end of the day and not *throbbing* by the time I get home.

CRYSTALS

Yup – you heard me. Crystals. Question all you want, but I feel better with them around and they're pretty to look at on my desk. Our whole profession is superstitious—so why not stack the deck in my favour? My favorites are black tourmaline and labradorite but use whatever you're drawn to. Except citrine...that one just brings trouble.

BREAKS

Breaks are a form of ritual. *Do not miss a break, if you have the option to take one!* Trust me. I guarantee, if someone asks you to go on break, and you decline, you *will not* get a break later. I used to put off going on break as I tried to tee up my assignment for success for the other person. In doing so, I missed countless breaks.

In a 12-hour shift there is never a good time to take a break. There will always be work waiting or someone needing attending. If *stat* orders are done, and you've at least seen your patients, take the break. Life is too short to burn yourself out by not eating or drinking or resting when you need to. There's a classic meme about being worried that your patient hasn't peed in four hours, yet you yourself haven't peed in ten plus hours. Where is the logic?

13 | HABITS AND RITUALS

JOURNAL PROMPTS

What do your shift routines and habits look like?
_____
_____

Is there a specific routine or ritual you have for certain tasks?
_____
_____

Do you have any rituals when it comes to the death of a patient?
_____
_____

What does your after-shift routine look like?
_____
_____

14 | NURSING SPECIALTIES AND THEIR ABILITIES

OVER THE YEARS I have worked with at least a hundred nurses in medicine, emergency, paediatrics, paediatric emergency, and recovery room (post anesthetic care unit). Every nurse is different but I've noticed how certain personality types fit better in the various departments. We've all seen the memes of the ER versus ICU nurse; med-surg versus the operating room and so on. In every job in the hospital setting, no day is the same and even less so for the ER. It's all about how we cope with chaos and then move on.

Here is a breakdown of the various departments and how I see personalities fitting in (described as a summary of personality traits that I feel fit within these diagnoses).

EMERGENCY ROOM

5% obsessive compulsive disorder (OCD), 95% undiagnosed Attention Deficit Hyperactive Disorder (ADHD).

Thrives on Chaos. Always looking for the next hit of adrenaline from saving a life.

OPERATING ROOM

100% OCD (Think Monica from Friends on steroids.)

Chaos isn't tolerated.

INTENSIVE CARE UNIT

90% OCD, 10% ADHD.

Doesn't thrive on chaos but tolerates it in small doses.

RECOVERY ROOM (POST ANESTHETIC CARE UNIT)

90% OCD, 5% ADHD, 5% Generalized Anxiety Disorder.

Chaos is an ever-looming threat, thus causing anxiety in those who are more OCD than ADHD.

MED-SURG

50% OCD, 50% ADHD.

It's a good mix of predictable and chaos depending on the patient ratio.

PAEDIATRICS

100% have the patience of a saint.

Can deal with the generalized anxiety of parents who must be pulled off the ceiling.

MENTAL HEALTH NURSES

They've already diagnosed themselves.

In all seriousness, thank you for what you do because I truly would not be able to.

LABOR AND DELIVERY

80% ADHD, 10% OCD.

Chaos is their bread and butter and THEN throw in the birth of a baby (or two, or three!).

PALLIATIVE CARE

100% compassion and kindness and care.

Angels walking among us.

To say that each of these groups of nurses have their own style and flair when it comes to organizing their day is an understatement. To be fair, I have mainly worked the ER, but when I travel to other areas of the hospital, I find that the way I organize my day in the ER, translates well when going elsewhere.

To find your niche, is to find your people.

15 | A DAY IN THE LIFE

COMING IN ON TIME

IN THE NURSING world, coming in "on time" means being ten to fifteen minutes early to be respectful of the person you're taking over for. Since it usually requires up to fifteen minutes to give a half decent report—I find I'll get a *better* report if I come in even earlier than the minimum. *Do not* be that person who barely makes it in the door (let alone ready for the report) at shift change. It won't make you popular, and quite frankly—it's disrespectful. You better believe everyone on the floor knows if you're chronically late. The effect will be that your colleagues will soon start to come in right at shift change for you, too. It's not much fun for anyone and trust me, coming in earlier puts you ahead of the game when it comes to the rest of your shift. It sets you up for success and is worth it, every time.

REPORT

As I said, coming in early affords me the time to get a great report from the shift before me. I feel more relaxed, and I usually end up being able to chat with my co-workers before rushing to get to report. Many times, as I receive the report, the shift before me will share an extremely important and ridiculously helpful hint or tip about the patient or their family that is useful to me as I go about my work. I am so thankful for this preparation. Trust me on this one.

GETTING ORGANIZED

Make sure to see the sickest patients first. If everyone (based on the report) seems to be okay, then I like to see patients in order of the rooms. It helps me to keep my patients straight and makes things go smoother when giving report at the end of shift. At the same time, I will go through my admitted patient charts to flag meds that are administered "off hours." I note antibiotics, or any other medications, not being given at a standard time. If I get busy, they can easily can be missed without taking extra organizational steps. The dreaded 6am medication is usually the first to be forgotten when trying to get ready to go home. You can also reconstitute medications that typically take forever to mix (e.g. Piperacillin/Tazocin or otherwise known in the USA as Zosyn) that's stable for twenty-four hours after being reconstituted). Mix in the normal saline or sterile water for the next twelve hours' worth of doses and then you can let them sit while you're doing other things. This save the rush to prepare the 6am dose because you forgot and don't want it to be late. We all know the medication takes *forever* to mix properly.

CLUSTERING VISITS, MEDICATIONS, AND INITIAL ASSESSMENTS

When I go in to assess my patients, I am usually doing a few things at the same time. I'll have their morning medications ready with their blood pressure meds in a separate cup so that as I check their vitals, (if their blood pressure is okay) I give them all their medications. As I assess a patient, I am doing vitals, giving their medications, adjusting the alarm volume on their cardiac monitors, (if they're on a monitor) changing the blood pressure cuff to go off every two to four hours depending on their orders and—after all this, asking if there is anything else they need while I'm there. This effectively cuts out four different in-and-out visits for the patient. This approach was originally started for those in isolation, so you were prepared with everything you needed and wouldn't waste time donning and doffing isolation gear multiple times.

This is easily the most effective way to save time and get things done ASAP. One of the rules I have for the ER is to use time in the best way possible because you never know when the shift is going to be flipped upside down. You don't want to be behind when that happens! Murphy's Law says that anything that can go wrong will, but if you can be prepared than it likely won't have as severe consequences. It's a total ER mindset because it' an unpredictable environment that changes day-to-day and minute-to-minute.

THE BELLS/ALARMS

For the love of all that is holy, if you have monitors at your patient bedsides, please try to turn down the volume! You can keep the central monitor volume loud, but there is no point in having a bedside monitor *blare* at every alarm so that after twenty-four hours, the patient has barely slept. This will make the patient more irritable. If you've spent any time in an ER as a patient or as a family member, you *know* what I'm talking about. As an extra note, if you're aware that your patient's normal heart rate sits in the fifties, please adjust your alarms. The whole room will thank you.

CHARTING

I chart soon after seeing a patient to prevent me from mixing up assessments. This way, if I forget the initial assessment by end of shift, I can go back to my charting and refresh my memory. Chart as often as you can. This is not a task to procrastinate on. You can potentially be hauled into court a year and a half after seeing a patient for one shift. I can almost guarantee you won't remember a single thing about the interaction, but your charting will!

Charting doesn't have to be long-winded, super descriptive or include everything that happened in your shift. The reality is that you have several times a day to capture what has transpired for each patient. A quick line or two on how the patient is doing will keep you on top of it. Check in on your patient, ask them if there is anything they need and reposition them. Then you can chart that the patient is: *Pink, warm and dry. Respirations free and easy.* These eight words form the basis of all my assessments. If this is *all* I have charted in two hours you can easily tell that the patient was perfusing well, breathing easily and most importantly, was alive at the time of assessment.

Those eight words also can change depending on patient status. Pink, warm and dry can be: pale, cool, mottled, pale or diaphoretic. Respirations free and easy can be: respirations laboured, shallow or patient is struggling to breathe. If you're having to modify your assessment of pink, warm and dry, respirations free and easy, then this also cues you to the fact that the patient's perfusion and respiratory status are not optimal, and the patient needs to be reassessed.

- Is there something that has changed?
- Have the vitals changed from what they were previously?
- Does the patient need PRN medication—be it pain medication, puffers, or something else?
- After your reassessment and attempt at PRN medications, has the patient improved?
- Do you need to call the doctor and update them as to the patient's condition?

These eight words are my everything. I use them countless times in a day and it's nothing if not simple. This is my greatest tip. If you chart often and if the assessment is truthful, you're golden. Know that a charting within an application like Epic and Meditech can change the time of the assessment, but the program will also document the actual time you are charting. This will come into play mainly in court situations. Charting as it happens, is not back-charting something that happened a few hours ago but was true as of the current time of charting. This will save your ass - trust me.

QUICK CHECK-INS

For a nurse, time can fly by during a shift but a patient will often be sitting in the same spot for twelve hours and only sees their nurse infrequently with hour-long stretches in between. This can make them feel like they are being overlooked. You and I know this isn't the case. You've got three to five *other* patients who also need to be seen and assessed including vitals and charting, but the person stuck in the corner with the curtains pulled doesn't feel this way. It helps if they have distraction—a book, their phone, a family member to talk to or even listening to the chaos surrounding them in their room. If the patient is normally an independent person who is experiencing pain, this can be an unsettling situation. Sometimes they get angry because they feel ignored or frustrated because they can't do much for themselves *and* they're bored. This is where a quick check-in can come in handy. It reminds you to pop in to see a patient and do a quick visual reassessment, and makes the patient feels seen.

15 | A DAY IN THE LIFE

Questions and needs also get taken care of before they fester, with the patient becoming more aggravated.

With this said I *know* that some shifts are crazy and sometimes the less urgent and quieter people tend to get ignored for longer stretches of time. If all you can manage is a quick round to pop your head in and ask if the patient needs anything, do it. And, make sure that their call bell is within reach. Your patients will be appreciative. I love patients who understand that there is more needing assistance than just them and so I go out of my way to not forget about them. They are usually the first people that I offer a warm blanket and water too. These simple things often get missed but can make a great impact. We've all heard the grateful ahhhh of a patient after a warm blanket is put on them. Then I'll hand over the largest glass of water I can get, with at least fifty percent ice, so that it stays colder longer. It's a small hack but totally worth the extra five seconds at the ice machine.

FEED THE PEOPLE

Yes, I know the longstanding joke about turkey "samiches" and the ER, but it's true. People tend to get extra ornery when they're hungry. Yes, I also understand that we don't feed those who are waiting for testing, could go to the OR *or* those who have been there a hot minute as well as not having access to a lot of food and saving it for those who will be admitted later in the day and not get a meal tray. Trust me when I say – if the patient can eat –feed them. If you're worried about nausea/vomiting, then explain this to the patient and hold off, but in most situations it makes your life easier to just feed your patients.

BATHROOMS

Always ask people if they need the bathroom. First thing in the morning, after their coffee, after lunch, after dinner and before bed. Think of how often *you* use the bathroom at home when you're not working. We're also probably pushing fluids if not running an IV for most patients. The easiest thing to do is offer a bathroom break, especially if your patient refuses to use the call bell. The bathroom check-in can be grouped with the quick check-in, giving you the opportunity to pair a free moment that you have with a patient need, thus decreasing their needs of you later in the shift. (Guaranteed to happen when you are swamped and can't help them.)

VITALS

In the ER, the standard of care is vitals every four hours. Obviously, this is for your stable, "probably leaving in a few hours" type of patient. If you think that something is going on, and your gut is telling you to pay attention, you can always do vitals more often and *chart them*! No one will ever fault you for paying *too much* attention to a patient. If you've put in the effort of doing vitals, (and thus quickly assessing your patient) chart it. Please, do me this favour. Do yourself this favour. Double check how often vitals are ordered by the doctor but to me, "vital signs routine" is every four hours.

THE FLUFF AND PUFF

Starting the day after getting report and going in to assess my people I also check to see if 1) they are in a brief or, 2) if their brief is wet. Yes, I know many people use the word diaper I prefer "brief". It's a respect thing. No one wants to hear their nurse yell to another nurse to get a diaper—especially if you're normally an independent person, and happen to get C.Diff and are too weak to get up and deal with the liquid diarrhea.

To "fluff and puff" someone is to make sure they're not sitting in a wet brief or left sitting on a bedpan (this has happened). Make sure their linen is dry and clean. Make sure the patient is sitting comfortably in the bed, and that their IV isn't leaking or gone interstitial.

I usually will do this at the beginning and end of my shift, just to make sure that I'm not leaving my patients in a disaster for someone else to come into. The last thing you want is to realize that someone has been sitting in a soaked brief for hours and now has skin breakdown.

REPORT

Congratulations! You've survived another twelve hours. I know you're tired and your brain has gone to mush but now you need to report off to the next nurse. There are a few key things that need to be included in a decent report that will tee up your co-worker for success for their shift.

- Past medical history—think big things like diabetes (thus blood sugar checks), dementia, sundowning, violence history
- Presenting complaint—why are they here *today*
- Alert and oriented or confused?
- At risk of a fall?
- Vital signs—is anything trending in the wrong direction or there were issues in the previous shift?
- Independent to go to bathroom or requires assistance?
- How things are going—improving, no change or getting worse? The nurse needs to know if the last twelve hours has gone in the wrong direction
- Consults to see—physio, occupational therapy, a specialist consult
- Testing that's pending—CT scan, MRI, angiogram, surgery that's planned to happen but hasn't happened yet
- MRP (Most Responsible Physician) – who you're calling if sh*t hits the fan
- Family member issues – is there someone who's been helpful, caring for this person? Or is there someone causing trouble when they visit?

"If you're breathing and not bleedin' it's a good day."

JOURNAL PROMPT

List extra items, specific to your workplace report.
_____
_____
_____
_____

16 | SO, YOUR PATIENT HAS DIED

I'M SORRY. It's that simple.

Some people like to try and compartmentalize the death of a patient and as always, everyone copes differently. Sometimes you can rationalize away the death of a patient — "they were older, it looks like they had a good life, and a family who loved them". Other times, (usually the times that are quick, violent, or unexpected) it's hard to make sense of the death of that person. It also hits differently depending on how long you knew the patient and their family. Sometimes, it's the grief and loss that you feel while watching the family grieve that hurts more than anything else.

Everyone reacts differently to loss and it's especially difficult at the beginning. Death can be a taboo topic. There is also the possibility of a new nurse not being exposed to a death in nursing school. This can make it that much more nerve-wracking. At least when you're a student no one expects much of you, other than to watch and learn. This allows you to become more comfortable with death and dying. Using your intuition can help you cope with the irrational. "Intuition and experience play a major role for nurses and for whom the emotional support of family caregivers is an essential aspect of the care they provide." Intuition can be used in so many ways, from helping your patient, to helping their caregiver, to helping yourself.

You learn many different lessons when someone dies while under your care. First, the "what if's" start. What if I'd done something differently? What if I'd called the doctor earlier? What if...what if...what if. You can drive yourself insane with the what ifs—especially with your first few patient deaths. The weirdness of having to remove everything off of someone (jewellery, clothes, tubes) and wrap them in a plastic bag naked never did sit well with me. To be honest, doing the toe tag also still bothers me and I will gladly pass off the task if someone else is willing to do it.

There are many parts of death that they don't teach in nursing school. They don't teach you how to comfort the family. They don't teach you how to gauge how quickly death is approaching for a palliative patient so you can give the family notice. They don't teach you how to deal with your *own* feelings about death and thus how it will shape the care you give up until the last moments.

You will have to dig deep, (really deep) to figure out how you feel about death, and if this death, this time, is melting away in your memory or sticking around in your head. Are you ruminating about the death? About the part you played in it? Are you asking questions that seem to go around and around with no real end? Do you have memories that are triggered by a certain room, smell, action, or type of patient you're dealing with? Sometimes a death will linger in your thoughts.

I've already told you about some of my rituals in dealing with death but maybe it's time to take a deeper look into them.

WARN THE FAMILY

If you have *any* suspicion that the patient is close to death (hours/days) *please* call the family. Give them the choice to come to the hospital or not. I have a certain speech that I tend to give families:

"Is this Mrs. _____ the daughter of Mrs. X."

"Yes."

"My name is Jenn and I'm a registered nurse in the emergency room where your mother is."

"Hi," they'll usually say, probably caught off guard a bit.

"I'm calling because your mother isn't doing so well. I'm worried that she's not going in the right direction and that her time may be coming. I wonder if there are family members who may want to come in and say goodbye before she dies." I say calmly, firmly and with as much clarity as I can.

"Oh," they say blankly.

"I hate to be the bearer of bad news, but your mother really isn't doing well, and I'd like to give you the opportunity to come in and spend some time with her. This is also a time to call family members if they are out of town. I worry that she's going to pass soon. If this was my mother, I would appreciate it if somebody would let me know that things aren't improving. Worse comes to worst, or better *comes to better, (your mother could turn a corner and ends up doing well) then at least it gives your family an opportunity to get an extra visit in. No one ever regrets coming in when there is the possibility that this may be the end. I always like to give people time when I feel like they have time. Sometimes people die faster than we anticipate, and we miss the opportunity to say goodbye."*

There. You've done it. You've given the family a choice—to come to the hospital or not. If they decide against it, that's their decision. Knowing that their loved one's death is approaching and giving someone the opportunity to say their goodbyes is a gift that can truly impact a family's grieving process. The golden rule applies here. Always remember to treat people like you'd want to be treated. That's why we call. If I can give people notice that their family member isn't doing well and it gives somebody the opportunity to come in and say their last goodbyes, it that makes my heart happy.

SUPPORTING FAMILY MEMBERS DURING THE DYING PROCESS

Everybody's grieving process is different, especially during the "actively" dying process. Families deal with the uncomfortable feelings surrounding death and dying in their own way. Some are hands on, wanting to be at the bedside. Other people are still very scared of death, and the process of dying. And that's *okay* too.

Figuring out how each family member is dealing with dying will let you know how you can best support them. If somebody is very hands-on, you can tell them how to watch for changes in their loved one's level of consciousness or pain responses so that they can ring the bell and let you know that the patient needs medication.

You can also reassure those who are not comfortable being at the bedside by letting the family know that it's *understandable* that they're not comfortable being at the bedside and that you know it's *normal* for them to be feeling overwhelmed. It's an uncomfortable process and some people aren't ready for it—let alone dealing with past traumas that may surface at the same time.

To watch someone die is extremely emotional, so provide lots of Kleenex. Make sure they've got water and that they are also taking time for themselves. If it's a slow dying process, families will need to rest and sometimes getting someone else's approval (i.e. yours!) to do so is the acceptance they need to hear. Sometimes it's not just the patient who's dying that you're taking care of, you're also taking care of their family.

MY DEATH RITUALS

- Closing the patients' eyes
- Removing all clothing, IV's, ET tube, catheter, ECG stickers, cardiac monitor stickers
- Talking to the patient like they're still there
- Removing jewellery and bagging it for family—charting what you took off and when it was given
- Rolling the patient and expecting a final exhale from their lungs
- Washing the blood/gore off the body to make it presentable
- Putting toe tag on
- Putting the body in the body bag
- Leaving underwear in place or putting a brief on to prevent spillage when the bowels let go
- Letting the soul out
- Being gentle with the body
- Wrapping the body while it's still warm makes everything easier for me personally
- Transport to morgue

MY FIRST PATIENT DEATH

My first patient death happened while I was a still a student on a maternity floor. I tell this story with permission from the family, with whom I have kept in touch with through the years. To Jason, Lucy and Grace—know that you're always in my thoughts when I try to remember where I've come from, and who I always want to be for my patients. This is for Sarah.

It was a regular day. Sarah and Jason had come in for Sarah's second c-section, planned and scheduled, just as her first had been. When inserting the IV during the preoperative phase, she had warned us that she had fainted the last time she got one. Sure, enough when we put in the IV, she passed out cold. It only took her a few minutes to recover and then she was fine.

The pregnancy had gone without a hitch. As the student, my role was to stay at the head of the bed and talk to the patient, keeping her calm and distracted until they could bring the husband into the room. As the sedation began, everything seemed to be going well. Yet, as the procedure started, Sarah began to say that she was going to die and that she was seeing God above her. Her comment stopped me in my tracks, the hairs still raise on my arm when I think about it.

I didn't understand what was happening. Suddenly everyone got quiet and the feeling in the room became very tense. As everyone worked behind the curtain Sarah told me about her cottage in the woods, how she loved that it was rustic and so far, removed from everything and everyone. She told me how it was lovely and how she was ready to go there. As a fourth-year student, I had no idea how to deal with this. I searched wildly for my preceptor, to tell her what was happening but I couldn't see her as there was a rush of extra people flooding into the room.

I didn't realize it, but when Sarah's baby was born they had to resuscitate her. I remember my patient looking over after the birth and wondering aloud why she couldn't hear her cry. Sarah looked where they were resuscitating her and called the baby's name out. "Lucy," she cooed, "come on little one, let me hear you." She spoke so softly, but I was able to hear her.

It was within the next moment that the baby cried out and the wave of relief washed over me.

"Okay," I thought aloud. "That's enough excitement for the day."

It was shortly after the baby was successfully resuscitated and were about to close my patient's C-section incision, that everything happened.

They didn't let Jason in and I wasn't sure why. Anesthesia was barking orders loudly over my head and I'm only understanding about half of what he's saying. The mood in the room turned from happy stress to anxiety and chaos. Before I knew it, my patients' blood pressure went high, then low, then high, then low. I had no idea what was happening, and Sarah keeps talking about how she's going to die and how she wants the baby to be called Lucy. She said she was ready to die and how she was so excited to meet God.

I told her everything was going to be fine, and I meant it. Everything was supposed to be fine.

But it wasn't to be. Moments after my patient heard her baby cry, she coded. This was my first code blue. My preceptor was the first to start compressions. She tells me to call the front and tell them that they've got a code blue and I'm gobsmacked, my feet frozen in place. She yells at me again to call the front and it's like I've been hit across the face. I jump into action and call the front to let them know what's going on.

CODE BLUE—MATERNITY—OR. I hear a loud overhead page begin, my heart quickening with each passing second.

CODE BLUE—MATERNITY—OR. The pager rings out again, this time seeming louder than before.

CODE BLUE—MATERNITY—OR. The last announcement blares out.

I have no idea what's happening. Everybody's yelling and the OR has collapsed into utter chaos. Five, ten, fifteen minutes go by, and I have no idea what's going to happen to the patient. It's all I can do to stay glued to the wall, pressing myself into it hoping that if I press hard enough, this nightmare will stop and I'll wake up. Seconds slip past. My heart pounds in my ears, the rushing sound starting to drown out the yelling. I'm getting lightheaded from the rush of activity, and I have no idea what to do.

We get a heartbeat back.

The whirlwind of activity slowed and I peeled myself from the wall, stepping forward to look at my patient again. I saw her lying with her eyes closed, motionless. Her long brown curly hair cascading off the OR table, like a waterfall. The tube down her throat is all I could focus on.

"I told her it was going to be okay," I stammered. The words ring in my ears, compounding the horrible way I was feeling. I promised her. *I promised her* it was going to be okay. The bile in my throat was rising, my mask suddenly feeling like it was preventing my breathing. I was going to be sick.

I hear a faint talking behind me and realize it's my preceptor trying to get my attention. "Jenn" she says. "Jenn," she puts a hand on my shoulder.

"Sorry Bernadette," I whisper.

"We're going to take her down to ICU if you'd like to come." She speaks ever so softly to me, treating me as if I'm about to fall apart. She's not wrong.

We packed up the multitude of IV pumps and transferred the patient to a stretcher. Her limp body swaying with the strong pull and push movements of the nurses. I stared at her eyes, closed now but I could've sworn they were open a second ago.

We walked through many hallways, each one becoming more bare and less aesthetically appealing. Near the end it feels like we're underground, in tunnels instead of hallways. The dark grey color of the concrete walls mirrored my own sullen mood. We transferred the patient to the ICU, and I hear my preceptor giving report. "Sudden cardiac arrest" and "not sure what the cause is" are muttered and I think they're the most unsettling words I've ever heard. I stay glued to the wall while report is being given, not wanting to get in the way in the busy ICU. I'm in a daze, unable to focus. All I can think is in that moment is "what the hell just happened?"

We eventually did get an answer.

Amniotic fluid embolism.

My preceptor and I make our way back to the maternity floor, not a word being said by either of us. It wasn't until we got back to the floor that my preceptor "turned back on," acting as if nothing had happened. I didn't know how she did it. She had been the one doing compressions. How was she able to switch gears like that? It was a skill that I hadn't yet learned, let alone mastered.

The event had happened first thing in the morning at 8am and lasted for about an hour and a half. After we got back to the floor, there was another laboring mom and there was no time to stop and process what had happened. A few hours went by and at roughly 1 pm the entire staff gathered into the nursing lounge. It was a tight fit, some people sitting, others standing. A proper looking woman in a pantsuit was waiting for us to file in. It was a full house and they closed the door. (I didn't even realize the lounge had a door!) The woman started by saying that the situation in the morning was unexpected, but that she was proud of how it was handled.

"*Situation?*" I thought "She had a name ..."

The woman continued to speak, but she'd lost me by referring to the code of this mom as a "situation." I slouch into the dark blue soft couch, happy to finally have a minute to stop and think.

"...they did everything they could," my ears burn. It was a phrase that I'd heard once or twice, and I started listening again as I hoped I'd heard incorrectly. "Unfortunately, at 12:22 this afternoon she died." A collective sigh escaped from everyone in the room and I see some of the nurses, as well as my preceptor, tear up.

Before I knew what I was doing, I said — "but I told her it was going to be okay. I *told* her it was going to be *okay*!" I didn't realize that my voice was getting louder. Tears were streaming down my face, staining my scrub top. "No, that couldn't have happened because I told her it was going to be *fine.*" My voice cracked as nurses began to surround me, holding me tight. I couldn't believe what I was hearing. The woman asked if anyone wanted to go home, and my preceptor volunteered that perhaps I should go, as I was in no condition to keep nursing that day.

It was easily a thirty-five-minute drive home and looking back I have no idea how I was able to safely drive home that day. All I remember is finally making it back to my childhood home, entering the house and crumpling onto the floor. My wails alerted my younger sister that something was wrong and she came barrelling down the long hallway to the top of the stairs to try to figure out what had happened.

I couldn't sleep that night. I tossed and turned, hearing the OR alarm bells and the shouting in my head. I kept thinking about the fact that I was the last person to talk to her—the last person to hear her speak, and to hear her last words. I realized that if I didn't write it down, no one would know that she had seen the baby and what she wanted that sweet little girl to be called. I got up in the early hours of the morning and wrote everything I could remember. I wrote fast and furiously as the memories came flooding back. I wrote and wrote. Once there were no more tears to cry and I had written everything I possibly could, I fell asleep for a few hours before having to get ready and go back to the unit.

16 | SO, YOUR PATIENT HAS DIED

Once again, we had an 8 am scheduled "routine" c-section. Looking back, I realize that I almost had a panic attack during it. The set-up was the same and it seemed that the new patient looked oddly like the one from the previous day. I kept having moments where I wasn't certain if I was seeing the new patient or having memories of the patient who had died. I'm not even sure if I breathed normally during the entire procedure. I was anticipating the alarms to start and the patient to deteriorate. My heart slammed into the wall of my chest the entire time. Then the baby was born, crying immediately. When I looked over, I saw that they'd let the patient's husband into the room. It was then that I also noticed that I was plastered against the wall in the exact same spot I'd been yesterday, my hands sweaty and not moving a muscle.

Thankfully, the c-section was quick and happened without incident. I'd overheard some nurses talking about how the baby from the previous day was doing quite well in the NICU. I thought about the husband who didn't get to say goodbye to his wife and I thought again about all the things that she had told me.

I went down to the gift shop and found two cute necklaces. One had a little ring on it that said faith, the other said strength. I bought two cards, one for the dad and one for the baby. In them, I wrote a message about how sorry I was for their losses. I had the piece of paper with me that I had written down the last words of the patient. In the babies' card, I shared that her mom had heard her cry and called her by her name. It was all I could do not to bawl while writing these cards, feeling the weight and responsibility of hearing somebody's last words. I went to the NICU and gave the cards, as well as the "faith" necklace to the dad. I kept the necklace that said strength.

Speaking with the family was overwhelming but oddly comforting at the same time. I got to see Lucy. She was beautiful and perfect, and I saw no trace of the trauma that had been the day before. It turned out that the patient's mother and father were there and were so grateful that I was able to give them the gift of their daughter's final words. I made sure to tell them that she wasn't scared, that she was going to their family cottage and knew that God was there. I went above and beyond because I felt *called* to go above and beyond. No one (in my mind) died in labour and delivery. It was a shock to me so I could only imagine what the family must have been going through. We cried a lot. We hugged and I left the NICU fully feeling the gravity of what had happened as it pertained to caring for not only the patient, but the entire family unit.

I wore that strength pendant for years. It was a symbol of the worst moment that I had seen and been a part of and a reminder of how I had overcome it to provide and care for the family after what was both the best and worst day of their lives.

My preceptor and I went to the funeral and were amazing by the number of family and friends present. It was in that moment that I realized the impact that one life can have on a community. It changed my perspective on many things from the role I play day in and day out as well as the role of family in the care of the patient. This patient stayed with me— my first trauma, my first code and my first death all in one. She was present whenever I would visit home up north and I always wondered if I would run into the family.

Turns out I did.

We were at a local Chinese restaurant during a winter break that I'd returned home to see my parents and siblings, taking a breather from the stress that was working as a nurse in the far North. Jason recognized me from across the room. I swear I felt like I knew he was there *even before* I saw him, as I can remember scanning the restaurant as we walked in. We couldn't help our tears as it had only been a few years since his wife had died. The baby and her older sister weren't there, but I got to see pictures of them.

In March a Facebook memory always pops up that I had posted the day *before* Sarah's death, about being excited to see my first c-section. It always takes me by surprise, causing me to pause and reflect again on that day, and that patient and her family and how much the experience changed me as not only a person but as a nurse as well.

If ever I am struggling with who I am as a nurse, I remember that at one point I had *so much* compassion and empathy. It gives me hope remembering that even in nursing school I got a life-changing lesson in compassion, empathy, and the role of family in the care of a patient. I embrace the naivety of my younger self and try my best to not be jaded by seeing people at the worst moments in their lives, day in and day out.

I give myself credit for getting this far and for keeping on when I could have walked away.

17 | SHADOW WORK

NOW THAT YOU'VE HEARD most of my traumas it's time to do a little introspection and shadow work for yourself to gauge where you are in the rollercoaster that is the trauma of working as a nurse.

Things are about to get uncomfortable. Take it easy on yourself and take as much time as you need to flesh out these ideas. One traumatic incident can cover *many* topics and there is no winning at who's most traumatized. Lord knows it's hard enough to do what we do without comparing traumas.

Take your time. It can be *a lot* to bring up the past and if you do this quickly or without truly focusing on the topics, it may catch you off guard. Some call it word vomit; I like to call it a brain dump. You dump out everything you're thinking about in the moment. Sometimes you can do a directed brain dump when you purposefully bring up painful memories or a traumatic situation by writing down everything you feel or can remember about it.

Don't think about what you're writing or dwell on how it makes you feel (right now). Just let it out and write it down.

JOURNAL PROMPTS

When thinking about a *minor* trauma(s) that have happened to you in your life/career, what do you think about? It may be something that irks you, but you don't dwell on it and it is easily put aside.

_____
_____
_____
_____

When thinking about a *major* trauma(s) in your life/career what comes to mind?

_____
_____
_____
_____

What feelings come up easily?

_____
_____
_____
_____

What feelings want to lurk in the back of your mind?

_____
_____
_____
_____

What was the *most* upsetting part?

_____
_____
_____
_____

17 | SHADOW WORK

What was the *least* upsetting part?
_____
_____
_____

What part haunts you?
_____
_____
_____

What part (if any) makes you smile or provides consolation?
_____
_____
_____

What part would you change if you could?
_____
_____
_____

What wouldn't you change?
_____
_____
_____

I need you to tell yourself (and begin to believe) that the outcome had nothing to do with what you personally did or didn't do. Some things are out of our control, and we're just witnesses to it.

I need you to forgive yourself and know that the situation was out of your control. You do not control who lives or dies. You can only do your part and the rest is out of your control.

People die.

In our line of work, sometimes a lot of people die, and some deaths are harder than others. You need to understand that nothing you did caused the situation. I know you know this. I know you want to believe it and I need you to.

I forgive you.

I forgive you for being *so damned hard* on yourself about every small detail. No one is perfect. No one person can have the answers. We do the *best* we can in the situation and then it's no longer up to us. I need you to let go of some of that pain. I know you can't let all of it go. Sometimes it needs to be chipped away in parts and pieces because the hole it's left in your soul is too big and too traumatic to come out in one sitting.

It's okay to heal. Tell yourself that it's okay to heal. You've held onto this pain for more than long enough.

- If you could tell the person who died that you were sorry and that you did all you could do, would you?
- If you could let the family know that you still carry that person with you, would you?
- Do you think that the family wants you to hurt like they do? What if the family has already come to peace with it but you're still carrying that pain?
- Was it a mistake that haunts you? Have you learned from it? Have you told others so that they don't make the same mistake?

Yes? Then, it's time to heal.

Give yourself some credit and kindness. No one is perfect. anyone who says they haven't made a medication error is either lying or the mistake wasn't brought to their attention. We do the best we can with the

17 | SHADOW WORK

support and staffing that we have in a day. You can't worl day in and day out without breaks. Saying yes to overtime may be stretching yourself thin and setting you up to fail. Being aware of the potential for lasting consequences relating to trauma is key. "Nurses with acute stress disorder may have trouble sleeping, worry constantly, and experience persistent negative thoughts about their role in the traumatic event." Nurses ignore our own emotions to protect against pain, but these emotions reappear over time and impact our lives. "Signs and symptoms of acute stress disorder may last for up to 30 days. If symptoms persist for more than a month, posttraumatic stress disorder (PTSD) is diagnosed."

It's okay to take care of yourself too. In fact, you *must* practice self-care to be able to sustain a career in nursing today. Don't be great at looking after everyone else but you? You shouldn't always come last.

Self-care is *not* selfish.

Say it again.

Self-care is *not* selfish.

One more time for the people in the back.

Self-care is not selfish.

18 | SELF-CARE ROUTINE

HERE ARE things that can help, when you start to feel burnout taking over. These may feel like common suggestions, and your personal preferences will always have a bigger impact on your own mental health vs. the generic solutions offered to you. One of the more "basic" recommendations is to have a routine that signals the end of your workday. This may include things like: taking a shower, reading a book, journaling, listening to your favorite music, calling a friend, watching your favorite TV show, or writing down things you were grateful for. These small things can be done quickly and easily to help signify the end of work helping you to transition into "off shift" mode.

Practicing regular self-care will help to build resilience, thus preventing burnout and potential long-term issues. "Nurses with passion or pride in their work and their profession are more likely to be resilient. On the contrary, nurses with lower resilience have higher levels of anxiety, depression and post-traumatic stress disorder" These rituals are key to prioritizing your heath, including physical, emotional and spiritual needs.

TAKE TIME OFF

Say *no* to the overtime. Period. Unless you are looking for extra income and the pickup won't completely screw with your sleep or plans.

Use banked time strategically to take time off. If you are full-time, there may be mental health days as well as sick days or holidays that can be used. Stop feeling guilting about taking a day just to focus on your own well-being. This can include doing *absolutely nothing*. There I said it.

Think about taking time off before you are so burnt out that you must take a leave of absence or stop working all together. Get ahead of the burnout. It's like pain gateway theory. Treat someone's pain when it's a 2-4/10 with Tylenol or Advil instead of letting the pain fester. If it gets out of hand and reaches an 8/10, then you can't manage it with over-the-counter medications, leaving you in need of serious help.

EXERCISE

List 3-4 shifts that you could potentially take off in the next 4 weeks. What would you do with a day off?

_____
_____
_____
_____

List 3-4 self-care appointments you could make with a day off. What self-care activity do you feel would have the most impact? Getting your hair or nails done? What about a massage? Why not use the benefits you pay into? What self-care activity would you love to get done *today*?

_____
_____
_____
_____

Is there an appointment that you've been putting off? Vehicle maintenance, a yearly physical, dental cleaning or something else? Would getting this appointment over with make you feel like you've accomplished something? What other appointments can't you find time for? It's time to adult today.

_____
_____
_____

Are you overwhelmed with house maintenance tasks? Can you break down how much an hour of your time is worth compared to hiring someone else to do it? Doing it yourself always seems like a great idea until you consider the time, effort and research you may need to put in to make the project work. Your "massive" project may be barely an hour's worth of work to a professional. Always ask, is this worth the time I'm spending on it?

18 | SELF-CARE ROUTINE

_____

_____

_____

Is there an activity that you really enjoy but have been putting off? Crafting, hiking, time spent alone in the wilderness? Is there an activity that you love that keeps getting put aside because there isn't enough time in the day? If you had your choice to spend a day doing your favorite activity, what would it be?

_____

_____

_____

_____

THERAPY

Yes, it's coming up again because I *whole-heartedly* believe that having someone you can vent to, who is a impartial third party, is amazing. Plus, they can help guide you in the areas you're struggling most with. I recommend my psychologist to anyone who will listen. She's helped me reframe thought processes that were really holding me back. She helped me to gain back my sanity. She is a saint.

If there was someone who you could talk to about the top three issues that cause you grief, would you? Knowing that those personal secrets were guarded, and you could be 100% honest and open, would you do it? What things come up now as issues causing you pain?

_____

_____

_____

_____

RELATIONSHIP EXPERT

In keeping with the therapy theme, do you think your relationship(s) could also use a tune-up? It could be the person you talk to about yourself, or it could be couples' counselling. There is nothing better than hashing out some longstanding argument with an impartial third party adding perspective. What things about your relationship could use addressing?

_____
_____
_____

SPIRITUALITY

I understand that everyone sees, and expresses, their spirituality differently. Does spirituality play a role in your life? Were you once an active member of a religious organization and now you've pulled away? What role did that play in your identity? Did your spirituality or religion help you to heal, or was it part of what tore you down? What does spirituality mean to you?

_____
_____
_____

During COVID, did friendships fall to the wayside because you were potentially a high-risk individual? Did it make you feel like an outcast? Did other people's opinion of your risk status change how you saw yourself? Did you isolate more than you potentially needed to, because you were worried you were going to be the reason someone got sick?

_____
_____
_____

Did/do you feel alone and unsupported? Do you feel like you're the one everyone relies on all the time? Do you feel like all the weight of the world rests on your shoulders and you have no on to share the burden with?

18 | SELF-CARE ROUTINE

Do you still have emotional baggage and trauma from COVID that you haven't dealt with?

Like everything and everyone you counted on at a time suddenly all those supports were withdrawn from you, and you were left to juggle it ALL, potentially alone, while being expected to show up to work and potentially put your life and the lives of your family in jeopardy because of COVID? Express how you really feel. Let it all go. There is no judgement.

_____
_____
_____
_____

19 | THE TOXIC CO-WORKER

USING YOUR GUT instincts to better understand the patients around you, can also (absolutely) be used to deal with your co-workers. A toxic co-worker is one who never seems to have anything nice to say; who continually complains about the workload and the patients. No matter how great the day, the toxic co-worker will put a damper on everyone else having fun, and seemingly has an inability to enjoy themselves. These people may also seem to push back against everything you do. Ask a question? They are the first to shut you down and make you feel silly. I consider this type of person to be an "energy vampire"— people who leave you feeling zapped of any happy emotions. Pay attention to your gut feelings. as these toxic people are ones to watch out for.

Starting work after graduation or even moving from one floor to another is always daunting. The change in skills and level of responsibility along with the worry about personality clashes is stressful. The only bonus to being a new graduate nurse, is if you've had very little or no experience with bullies. If bad behaviour isn't directed at you, it's easy to shrug off and explain the behaviour as "just having a bad day," or "they're feeling overworked" or maybe there is family issues?

First, thank you for thinking outside the box and giving your co-worker the benefit of the doubt. Giving that person the opportunity to explain their behaviour before going straight to management with concerns can be one way to nip bad behaviour in the bud. Take that person aside and privately if they're okay and ask about the behaviour. This takes a lot of courage if you don't really know the person but could stop the behaviour in it's tracks. Maybe this person just needs a bit of support and is feeling overwhelmed and happened to snap. However, if it is a repeating pattern there is more than likely behaviour that can become bullying behaviour. One of those reasons for bad behavior is truly one nurse to another and still needs to be addressed so as not to become a habit of someone's.

"Bullying is a negative behavior directed toward a victim, a fellow employee, that occurs in the workplace. It can encompass nonverbal behaviors, such as rolling eyes, ignoring a fellow employee, or walking away when approached. Verbal behaviors include snide comments, derogatory comments, yelling, or teasing."

It might be that someone just needs to take this person aside and ask them if they're okay. Offering a safe space to talk can help, but it does take a lot of confidence to be able to ask a stranger if they're alright. Bullying in nursing is a well-known phenomenon and has a longstanding history. Of all the skills and knowledge that were seemingly skipped during nursing school; bullying was a topic that was well-covered. If someone has singled you out and is actively making your life a living hell, that's another story.

In my thirteen-year career, I've seen countless incidences of bullying and been on the receiving end of bullying by four different nurses. Those were the targeted incidences, and does not include all the comments and backhanded "compliments" made by a multitude of nurses through the years. I am including my stories so you can watch out for the telltale signs that you're being bullied and the various ways that it happens.

There are long-term mental side effects as well as overall health effects when you are bullied. "Higher incidence of bullying was associated with lower physical health scores and lower mental health scores. Nurses who are bullied at work experience lower physical and mental health, which can decrease the nurses' quality of life and impede their ability to deliver safe, effective patient care."

There are many facets to bullying and various degrees of it.

- Sometimes it's insidious—such as gossiping behind your back rather than actual face-to-face interactions.
- Another scenario is being purposefully set-up to fail in the form of a nursing assignment that is exponentially heavier than any other assignment.
- Sarcastic comments, making you question your nursing abilities
- Yelling at you in front of a room full of patients.

19 | THE TOXIC CO-WORKER

I have experienced all of these situations and they're all awful. They make you anxious to go to work because you don't know if that bullying person will be there. You wonder if today the day will be the day that you that you end up—not just crying at work—but crying *in front of them*. "Nurses who are bullied at work experience lower physical and mental health, which can decrease the nurses' quality of life and impede their ability to deliver safe, effective patient care." The list of negative side effects of bullying is well-documented and has been studied to death, yet it continues to be a pervasive theme in nursing regardless of unit, hospital, or shift. The likelihood of nurses experiencing or witnessing bullying during their career's ranges from 17% to over 90%. This statistic (as staggering as it sounds) seems bang on to me. I don't think I've had one job where if I wasn't the subject of the bullying, then I at least witnessed someone else being bullied. I used to think emergency nursing was just callous and rough and tumble. It turns out that the paediatric nurses were some of the most toxic people I've ever come across, but we'll get to that in just a bit.

Thus far, the only good thing to come out of being bullied is the fact that I now *refuse* to let it happen to anyone else on my watch. For me, bullying is the ultimate "knife in the back" that you'd least expect in a profession with a mandate of caring for people. "Workplace bullying is a situation when an ongoing attempt is made to force a person out of their job by gathering people— either with or without their own approval— around another person to perform malevolent actions, make insinuations, mock them and lower the person's social standing, and create an aggressive atmosphere." Bullying in nursing is somehow so pervasive that when a new person is orientated to the unit, there can be warnings about certain people included in an orientation. Again, this happened to me. It still shocks me because I would have *never* expected such behaviour and yet, it did after I'd already been in one *extremely* toxic environment and a second one slightly less so. I was so done with taking everyone else's bullshit.

As I share my personal bullying stories, please know that they still produce an incredible amount of anxiety for me. So much so, that my hands are already shaking as I type. The thought of reliving the worst moments in my life obviously don't fill me with any sort of joy. I'll go in order of severity to show you how I started and how, after the second and third instances of bullying, I was finally able to start standing up for myself.

No one should *ever* be made to feel the things I felt, especially to the extent of thinking about suicide. Reach out for help if you find these stories triggering. I made the mistake of waiting too long, thinking that I was "too strong" for medications and therapy. Please don't suffer in silence, especially *from a job*. I support your decision to leave that workplace *1000%*. You will not be the first or last to leave a unit because of toxic behaviour. If I've learned anything from the last thirteen years, it's that there is *always* another job or unit to go to.

Make your mental health a priority, because the bully will usually not stop until they get you to crack.

20 | THE MOST TOXIC PLACE I'VE EVER WORKED

TO SAY THAT I STILL have moments of panic and fear thinking about this workplace is an understatement. It was a job that caused me *years* of trauma. It was in a small town—barely a blip on the map—that I landed in the most toxic workplace I've ever worked.

It was my first hospital job, and I was just so new I *shone* green. I was excited and more than ready to get my nursing career underway. I don't know what it was about me that my supervisor didn't like but it seemed like she couldn't stand me from the moment I walked through the door. She worked eight-hour dayshifts, oversaw the schedule and was the queen bee of that unit.

I had finished orientation. The hospital only had one Registered Nurse (RN) for the emergency department and one RN for the floor, with two Registered Practical Nurses (RPN) for support. What that meant for me as a brand-new nurse was that I would get a quick orientation to both the floor and the ER and was expected to be proficient in both. The plan was to always have me working with a more experienced RN so that if I needed help, someone would be there for guidance. I was part-time and therefore not in a rotation. My supervisor was 100% in charge of my schedule.

It started with my being booked mostly nights which didn't bother me. Then, it quickly turned into being scheduled for quick turn arounds (I would work a night shift, get off the next morning at 7:30, go to bed and try to sleep until 3ish because I was scheduled to work a dayshift the next day). In our union contract this technically wasn't allowed because of the time it takes to bounce back from nights to days, but I didn't say anything because I was new. I didn't want to rock the boat and figured it was normal for new grads to "pay their dues". I wasn't the only new grad put in this situation, but I was the one it happened to the most.

After I started working on my own, the comments started. My supervisor would make little jabs about how I did or didn't do something. Being naive, I thought she was trying to be helpful! She may not have been saying it tactfully, but again I was new and chose to see the optimistic side of it. The little comments quickly turned into flat out criticisms of whatever I was doing. At first the comments were made out of earshot of the patients and other nurses, but this didn't last. In no time I was being criticized in front of co-workers and then in front of my patients too. I was mortified and it got to the point where I purposefully begam to avoid her—which in a hospital with only a teeny tiny ER and 14 or so beds, was *very* hard to do.

I switched into more nights and weekends to avoid being in the building at the same time as the Queen Bee. I was told by other co-workers that she always had an issue with someone, this was just my turn. As I look back, the idea of this still makes me uncomfortable. The fact that she did this to everyone, not just me, was somehow supposed to make me feel better about the abuse I was taking?

A few weeks went by, and the behaviour escalated. I started to worry about going into work, wondering what would happen that day and how upset I'd be when I got home. It was at this point that I started to drink regularly, numbing my feelings of unworthiness, fear, and anxiety. I had never been much of a drinker, and used it solely as a coping mechanism. After a rough shift, I would call my (now) husband and ask him to have a bottle of wine and a glass ready when I walked in the door.

This hospital itself was so small, that the smallest of nightshift duties were taken *very* seriously and if nightshift tasks weren't done, it tended to be a much bigger deal to dayshift than it would've been in any other hospital. Things like making sure there were extra pieces of paper, and doctors' orders in the charts ready for dayshift was a *big* deal. I'm telling you—I'd be brought into the boss's office for a conversation about paper supplies, in a nursing station that barley held three chairs. The paper was so close to everyone that it would have taken two seconds to grab some out of the drawer. Everything, no matter how small, was made into a big deal. So, when I made my first medication error within my probation period, it was a *disaster*.

20 | THE MOST TOXIC PLACE I'VE EVER WORKED

THE STORY

It was a bright and sunny dayshift, the afternoon sun shining through the large glass door that led into the small ER. I was working in emergency portion and it was one of my first shifts alone in the ER after orientation period, having the majority of the shifts prior being on the medical floor. It had been a slow day as usual. I had a patient who was experiencing a chronic cough and my doctor ordered hycodan (morphine) syrup. I wasn't very familiar with narcotic cough syrup, so I took a few minutes before drawing it up to look it up online. It was after that quick check that my doctor asked me to get 40 millilitres of the syrup.

I verbally confirmed the dose. "You said 40ml of hycodan syrup, right? I asked.

"Yes," she said and continued writing on the patient's chart, her head bowed in concentration as she continued to scribble her patient notes on the chart.

I poured the thick, pinky red syrup into two medication cups as 40 ml's wouldn't fit into one alone. I passed the small plastic cups to the patient and instructed her to drink both. The patient looked at the medications color, raising an eyebrow at the shockingly bright color of it.

"Cheers," she said and tipped back the first cup. Two to three seconds went by and she drank the second tiny cup of medication. It was at that time that the doctor poked her head around and asked if I had given 40 mgs of syrup or 40 mls of syrup. I had said that I gave 40 mls as ordered by her.

She stopped and looked at me. "No, I meant 40mg." She said coolly.

My heart had never dropped in my chest so hard and so fast. I began to panic because I'd never made a medication error before. I called up to the floor to talk to the other nurse and she came down to help me as I felt lost and unsure of what to do next. We started an IV to give the patient fluids. The active ingredient in hycodan syrup is morphine so thankfully the patient's only symptom after the medication error was becoming a little drowsy. But I was a wreck.

I remember slipping into the tiny bathroom across the hall from the ER and crumpling to the floor. My breaths were ragged and shallow. I had no control over what my body was doing or how it was reacting to the stress of this situation. Not only had I made a medication error, but I felt so *guilty* about potentially hurting a patient. I was overwhelmed that I'd made the error and didn't know what else to do. Thankfully my partner saw that I was a disaster and shoo'd me away as I tried to return to the ER without fully shutting down my emotions. She started the IV, kept an eye on the patient and continued to chart. In all honesty, she saved my ass in that scenario —keeping her cool as I was losing mine.

After a few short hours the patient was alert enough to go home. I profusely apologized to the patient and thankfully she was wonderful about the whole thing. She told me not to worry and that she was okay and not hurt in the slightest. She comforted *me* during one of the lowest points in my short career. She left later that day, walking out under her own power, like nothing had happened. She joked that the cough was taken care of. I tried to laugh at the joke but my guts were still too on edge.

After the patient left, I went to look for my Director of Nursing to inform him of what had happened. I passed by the doctor's lounge and as I did so, the doctor I'd been working with called me in. She was sitting on an old couch that had clearly seen better days. It sagged where she sat in the middle of it, and she asked me to sit beside her. I sat down, hands in my lap as they continued to sweat profusely even hours after the incident had happened.

"I just wanted to say that I'm sorry I made that medication error," the young doctor blurted out. She too was wringing her hands in her lap. I was stunned. I just looked at her thinking that it had been my error in not recognizing the dosage wasn't being ordered the correct way.

"Oh...hey, I mean...I thought you said 40 ml's, but...ugh...I...I should have caught it too" I stammered, words failing me in the moment. I'd only been out of school a few months and I still felt like the doctors were in a league above me. There was a power dynamic that ebbed and flowed between the doctors and nurses at the hospital.

"No, it's okay" she said. "It was my error too; we just have to be a bit more careful next time." She looked to me and smiled weakly. I nodded and stood up, moving closer to the door, feeling uncomfortable in the sacred "doctors' space" that was the doctor's lounge. As I stepped into the hallway, I felt better knowing that the mistake was no longer my own and

20 | THE MOST TOXIC PLACE I'VE EVER WORKED

that the doctor and I were on the same page about what had happened. It made updating my Director of Nursing feel so much easier.

I was open and honest about what happened, and let him know that the doctor and I had already spoken and agreed about what had happened. I felt more empowered as I walked into his office and explained the situation. He suggested that I go home, and I said that was fine. I wanted to think about everything that happened. Things would be better by tomorrow.

Man was I wrong.

The next day I was pulled into the director of nurse's office so quickly my head spun. He explained that they had started an investigation and wanted to get my recollection of everything that had happened. I was extremely upset to have to delve into those emotions again, but tried to recount everything to the best of my best ability. I told him everything I could remember. It felt like he loomed over me as he was easily over six feet tall and had a slight frame. His face relayed concern and he didn't say a word as my words tumbled out. I explained that thankfully the patient was fine, and returned home with no adverse effects. As his gaze bored into mine, I repeated that I had apologized profusely to the patient before leaving and that she graciously told me not to worry about it. We sat there in silence.

I reminded him that I'd spoken with the doctor and that she agreed that she too had a role in the medication error. I was shaking in that uncomfortable chair. He sat back, keeping his hands clasped and crossing one leg over the top of the other. He seemed to be quietly contemplating. I asked if I could return to the floor to finish listening to report. It was then that he informed me that I would be on paid leave until the investigation concluded. I asked about my patients, and was told that they had replaced me the day before. He showed me the door.

I drove home in utter shock. It wasn't even 8 am. The cold air slapped me in the face as I finally reached home, got out of my car and walked into the house. Then the tears started to fall.

I still felt awful, but now I had a bigger thing to worry about. Certainly, I'd made an error. I wasn't hiding it. I took full responsibility. I was confused about the "investigation." Why wasn't it already settled? Again, I drank—to numb the pain, confusion, and fear about what the hell was going on. It was all I could do to stay home that day. How long was the investigation going to take? Thankfully my husband had a full-time job, and the bills weren't a worry but what if…. Stop thinking like that, I told myself. It was a simple error that both the doctor and I took responsibility for. It wouldn't take long to sort out.

Within a few days, I was called back into the director of nurse's office. I was handed a letter of termination.

What. The actual. Fuck!

I was screaming internally, the ringing in my ears so loud that I could barely focus on what was being said. "Someone came forward with a list of concerns about your practice," he stated. "We've decided that the best course of action is to let you go." The words cut me with each syllable.

I thought I was going to throw up and looked feverishly around the room for a garbage can. "But, the doctor talked to me yesterday…" I stammered it out. "She and I talked, about how this was both our mistake. We agreed. This was *both* our mistake." The words tumbled out of my mouth. "Did you talk to her?" I ask, my eyes wide with fear.

"Yes, we talked with her. She said she wrote the order as 40mg's not 40 ml's. She said it was your error." he straightened his back to distance himself from the puddle of emotions that I was becoming.

She lied. She *lied*! I felt the anger rising in my chest. I'm done. With one sentence, all hope I had of coming back from this disappeared. The doctor lied, preferring to sink me and my career. She offered me up like a sacrificial lamb to slaughter, taking absolutely no responsibility for what had happened.

The tears. Those damned tears started again. My termination letter became more damp with each passing minute. Again, my director offered no condolences, no words of comfort. He just stood and waved his arm at the door, signaling that I was to leave his office.

The devastation was real. Doubt, fear and anxiety overwhelmed me. I felt I had no control over what had just happened. The loss of my innocence and trust in others that day was monumental. I could no longer trust *anyone*. I went home and even though it was early morning, started to drink. Who was I without being a nurse? How will I work? How will I tell my parents? With each question came the overwhelming need not to

20 | THE MOST TOXIC PLACE I'VE EVER WORKED

feel numb. I drank and I drank. Days went by until I was so hungover that I needed to stop drinking because I was in too much pain. With being sober came the anger and that turned out to be my saving grace.

The doctor had *lied*.

I thought about the other things my director said. Who had concerns about my practice? Was I even able to be fired while part of the nursing union? My anger kept me sober.

Technically, because I was still on probation when the director fired me, he didn't have to provide me or my union with any reason for termination. However, he did cite cause which gave the union an "in" to fight the termination. I took full responsibility for the medication error, but I wanted to see the list of "practice concerns" and I wanted to see who had made the complaint. I was suspicious, wondering if my bullying nursing supervisor was somehow involved. It took a few weeks to build my case and get the grievance filed, but the union was ready to fight and so was I.

The meetings with the union and the Director to fight for my job were some of the hardest moments that I've ever dealt with. After much deliberation and a few weeks of back-and-forth, it was decided that I would get my job back but would have to restart the 525 hours of probation, with the added stipulation that I could (again) be fired at any time for no cause and that would be the end of it.

I had my job back, but the rumours about me had started. In such a small-town, rumours travel faster than wildfire and suddenly, I was the black sheep nurse who had been fired. Suddenly all the friends that I thought I had, disappeared. No one would visit my house and no one was returning my phone calls. I felt very alone and it was devastating. I already felt at a disadvantage because it wasn't my hometown, and no one really knew me. I was a "southerner" who didn't belong and I sure as hell felt like that while working through the negotiations with the hospital. The looks I got when I went out to the grocery store were not even veiled and people would stop talking and start whispering when I passed by. It was isolating and degrading, and I felt the lowest I've ever felt. Before that point I'd never once had mental health issues or thoughts about killing myself, but that town brought out the absolute worst in me. There was a moment driving back to the town after a visit with my parents that I wondered if I should just drive my truck into the jagged rock and make it easier on everyone. The thought was thankfully short-lived but left a permanent mark on my spirit.

It took months before I was ready to return to the hospital to "start over" and let me tell you the daily anxiety that I was battling was more than I ever want anyone else to face. Truthfully, I should've been medicated with either anti-anxiety meds or anti-depressants but I fought to stay off them. I don't know why. Everyone kept telling me how strong I was and that I didn't need medication...but, I did. I needed help and I should've been strong enough to ask. A mistrust of all the doctors I worked with—including my family doctor—was engrained deep. They all must've heard that I was fired, they all must've heard their colleague's version of "my" mistake. How could they trust me after something like that? How could I trust them?

On my first day back to work you could hear a pin drop in report. No one looked directly at me and I could hear the hushed whispers of everybody talking behind my back. In those moments, I knew I was alone. There was no support, there were no friendships —only cattiness and disrespect. It was no longer just a supervisor who was against me, it was everybody I worked with. Everything I did had to be perfect. Everything I did had to be exact. There was no room for error.

I dreaded working. I was filled with dread every minute leading up to work and started a countdown to the end of my probation. I didn't mention it though, I was afraid that if they knew time was running out, that they would again fire me without cause.

Five hundred and twenty-five hours. Counted down until the very last minute.

I finished my probation. I was kind of shocked that everyone let it happen. I became a permanent part-time staff, but the damage was done. I knew I was alone in whatever struggles I would face, that nobody would have my back if I messed up and that no one was my friend. To tell you that I had moments of panic before walking into that door every single day is to minimize the trauma that returning to that toxic workplace really was. I dreamt of leaving of walking away and leaving it in my past but I didn't do it for five more years.

20 | THE MOST TOXIC PLACE I'VE EVER WORKED

Five years. Five years of stress and panic and worry and faking that everything was fine. Five years of faked niceties. Five years of overactive stress and panic. Five years of daily pain and suffering. Five years of showing up every day and pushing down my true feelings about that hospital and its staff. Five years of fake smiles, fake friendships and so much drama and gossip that those years could be covered in their own book.

People told me I was strong for going back. Truly, I felt like I had no other option. There wasn't a lot of work for nurses in that town and my husband and I had just moved in together. I wanted to continue that relationship—it was the only thing that kept me going for a long, long, *long* time. The way I know that the workplace was toxic is that I actually considered leaving my husband just so that I wouldn't have to go back to that workplace. That relationship was my saviour. When no one else knew how badly I was struggling, he was there, and he did.

After I finished my probation, it was spite that kept me going. *Pure* spite. It became easier to pretend like nothing had happened. I went day by day. We used to joke about me picking up my little black cloud when I walked into the hospital and then leaving it behind when I went home. Of course, that was never the case. I promised myself that I would be the most educated nurse to ever walk out of that hospital. I dreamt of quitting, of writing a resignation letter and of all the various ways I could quit. Would I be professional? Would I yell or scream or call out those who had hurt me along the way?

For five years I didn't rock the boat but every single day was a struggle. Every time that my supervisor could put in a cutting word, she did. Every time she could make me feel like I was two inches tall she would. The gossiping, the pitting people against me was never ending but still I held my head as high as I could during those moments. Don't misunderstand. I *wanted* her to get back some of what she was giving but there was no point to it. A group of us sat down one night shift and calculated that over 20 years she had pushed at least 12 nurses out of the hospital.

In a town of 5,000 that was a big number and yet not in the least surprising.

21 | MY INTRODUCTION TO NURSING

I HAD A DAYDREAM about applying to jobs back in Southern Ontario. Various scenarios played out in my mind. The singular thought about getting to say the words "I quit" became a sort of obsession. My husband and I would have long conversations about how unhappy I was and how one day my dream would become reality. Then, one *glorious* morning, my husband called and uttered the most wonderful seven words that I'd heard in a longest time. I got the job. You. Can. Quit.

It started with an argument and him saying that I was free to apply to jobs if I was unhappy. I may have taken the sentiment a little far and *littered* the internet with my resume. It wasn't long before calls for interviews started, with job offers quickly following. I was excited, but there was no way we could afford to move without my husband having a full-time job as well. Months went by. He just couldn't seem to find a job in his niche market. I wondered if I would be stuck in the small-town hospital for the rest of my life. After five months of waiting and wondering if a job would ever become available, I started sinking into sadness again.

Then it finally happened and I was delirious. I asked him multiple times to repeat himself. He kindly said again that yes, I could quit and that he was happy that I was happy. It was all I could do *not* to scream at the top of my lungs. My hands shook with anticipation and excitement, and I felt like I could throw up all the anxiety that I had been holding in my gut for five years. It was over. Done. No more having to pretend like I was happy. No being fake. I was free. I would start over and never utter the word "fired" ever again. I could be and do whatever I wanted. I don't remember typing up my resignation. I didn't remember printing it out. I don't even remember getting dressed or driving over to the hospital. You better believe my petty ass somehow was aware enough to put on the exact same outfit that I interviewed in.

Picture me in white kitten heels, a brilliant white blazer and bright white knee length skirt, my bright cornflower blue top peeking through. The look that I must've had on my face walking into the hospital that day? I can't even imagine. I marched into that building like I was someone else—someone who hadn't been beaten down and held against my will for five years. I wasn't the same meek, small, quiet person that they all knew. Now I was confident, feeling so much like my prior self, before I made myself smaller to fit inside their box. I can still hear the click clacks of my white kitten heels on the cheap, faded linoleum as I began looking for my two targets.

I turned towards the medical floor, peering into every office on the way. I soon gained the attention of my fellow co-workers. "Wow!" They exclaimed. "How come you're dressed to kill?"

"I'll tell you in a minute" I say, winking at them and enjoying the fact that they have no idea what's about to happen. Even I was unsure what I was going to say and do. I find the director of nursing. He comes out of the office, and I notice that I no longer find his tall stature intimidating. I look at him with resentment and can feel the excitement bubbling up inside. The anxiety I was so used to feeling, that I associated with this building, was about to be replaced with my own brand of justice. He sees me and his face dropped, ever so slightly, his features losing the confidence they once had. I think that somehow, he knows that he no longer has control over me or my career. I open my mouth to speak, and barely recognize the sharp tone that comes out.

"Do you have a minute?" I ask, tilting my head ever so slightly, a slight smile curling on my lips. (As I write this, I admit that I must've seemed slightly deranged).

'Sure." He answers quickly and makes his way towards his small office across the hall. I follow him in. "What can I help you with today?" He asks.

"Here's my resignation" I say, "and this is my two weeks' notice." I try and say it as politely as I can. I may be more than excited to quit, but there is a part of me who wants to try and take the high road and be professional. I pass him my letter of resignation, my hands shaking with delight.

"Oh," he says taken aback "this is a surprise."

21 | MY INTRODUCTION TO NURSING

It takes all my effort to supress the jolt of wry laughter that's bubbling in my gut. How could he think this was not going to happen? Did he truly think I would take the constant belittling, mistreatment and terrorizing that happened damn near every shift? He couldn't be that daft. Unless he thought I would just take it. Unless he thought I would take it for an entire career, like others had. Fuck that.

Instead, I sit, cross my legs like a lady and for the last time ever, pretend to give a shit about what this guy is talking about. He drones on about how he's blindsided by my decision and goes on to say he's proud of me. *Proud of me.* I sat there, head nodding, hands holding onto one another to remind me to not say anything I'd regret later. I forced a weak smile like the pain and anguish of the last years hadn't happened—like quitting this job wasn't the one thing I was more excited to do than anything else. Ever.

As politely as I can, I tell him that no matter what the outcome has been, that this little hospital had been my introduction to emergency nursing. I tell him we are moving down south as we both have gotten jobs. Sure, enough when he asks where we're moving too it turns out that we're moving to his hometown. I try and stay focused as we *very politely* talk about the growing experiences that I've had and how it was *quite* an education. After a handshake and my very last fake smile, I walk out into the hallway to track down my supervisor to give her the glorious news of my resignation.

As I approach the nursing station, I see a collection of the dayshift nursing staff. They snap to attention to hear the news that I said I would share. "I quit." I said puffing out my chest, smile broad. "I just put in my two weeks' notice."

The round of "congratulations" and "way to go" are uttered half-heartedly as I know a few of them wished they had the option to leave as well. I answer a few questions before reminding myself that I was on a mission but before I take a step towards my nursing supervisors office, she comes scuttling out. Her short brown hair swooped across her forehead in what is now known as the typical Karen haircut. I try to catch her eye through the nursing station glass but she's moving fast. My smile broadens and I'm giddy to tell her that I quit. She passes by me without making eye contact.

I call out, "Hey, do you have a minute?"

Without looking up she says, "Yep, you're quitting. Okay," and strode past acting as if I didn't exist.

It was in that moment that I realized I was never going to get the apology that I wanted. It was also in that moment that I realized that it no longer mattered.

I had accepted that I would never fit in. The people pleasing part of me now seems more of a trauma response than I realized before that point. There wasn't any point in sticking around the hospital any more than I had to. I opening the glass door on my way out, having to put a bit of my weight into it to get the door to open. As I push forward, I am released out into the bright, sweet sunshine of the day and my senses are overwhelmed. The air smells sweeter. I feel a brush of breeze against my face and I feel more at peace than I have in a very long time. I take a moment to savor my new freedom.

The next two weeks flew by. Finally having the freedom to say and do whatever I wanted while at work was very tempting. I only had a dayshift or two in that time and all I could do was smile and laugh as my supervisor continued to look as miserable as ever. It was no longer my concern. In a final act of control and manipulation, my supervisor cancelled my last three shifts, ending my last week suddenly and without cause and I couldn't have cared less.

My last day was not even celebrated because no one knew that it was going to be my last day (except for my supervisor). There was no goodbye party, no farewell potluck and no get-together for drinks. The closest thing to a celebration happened because I was leaving during nursing week. The hospital committee had rented a karaoke machine in the Legion Hall for an evening. There were only been three or four people in the Legion by the time I arrived and none of them were even nurses. I got drunk. So. Very. Drunk. *Little Bird* by Annie Lennox was always a favorite of mine and decided that it was an appropriate going away song. What I happened to forget in my drunken stupor was just how long the song was and just how high the notes were. I didn't care and without an ounce of shame, I belted out the song!

I was done, I was free, and I got to get out of there alive.

22 | BULLY ENCOUNTER #2

MY SECOND BULLYING ENCOUNTER was after attempting to find my "dream job." My husband had been being head hunted by a hospital system and I found myself in the position of also wanting to move into the same organisation. The deal between my husband and I was that if I should get my dream job we could move from where we were to the next town over. It took a little bit of time, but I finally got a part-time position in what I thought was going to be the emergency department of my dreams. It started out innocently enough (as it usually does) my preceptor seem to be cool, fun, and easy going to start but it quickly became pretty evident that she was part of a horrible clique. It seemed to me that this emergency department was very particular about the things that they did and how they did them. IV insertions being a cornerstone of the differences between this emergency department and the others I had worked in. The nurses didn't seem to have as many medical directives to work with when patients came in limiting the number of interventions that could be done before the Doctor saw the patient, thus slowing down the process of getting patients ready for the Doctor to see them and potentially have all the information they needed for a swift discharge home. The unit was very specific about how everything had to be done a very certain way and if it wasn't done that way then it was frowned upon. Regardless of how small the task seemed to be (think the way an IV is secured). It didn't necessarily matter if the way I did it still got the job done, but it seemed the fact that I was suggesting a different way seemed to be the main problem.

Trust me I tried not to be that person to say, "oh well at my last job we did it this way" or "at my last job we did it that way." I was mindful of that those types of sayings never come across well and yet I still seemed to rub a select few people the wrong way. Slowly the comments and behaviours started. They weren't often actually directed at me, but I could tell that they were being said. There were multiple occasions of a certain charge nurse deciding to put inappropriate patients into my area and watching what happened. Kind of like a sink or swim scenario. Sadly, the ER is normally awful when it comes to this behaviour, we tend to want to put people in positions to see if they can swim or if they're just going to sink and maybe the ER isn't for them. I understand this is deplorable behaviour and we need to teach people the ways of the ER as it is vastly different from any other unit regarding flow and potential for disaster.

Of course, as charge she had the ability to delegate which patients went where and it seemed often that I would get the heavier sicker patients compared to everybody else. I noticed, my coworkers noticed, and even my doctors noticed that my section of the ER would be full when everybody else had maybe one patient when she was charge nurse. It wasn't long before one of my fast friends in that ER, a healthcare aide took me aside and asked me if I had noticed what had been happening. I am so thankful for her to have the ability to make sure that somebody was okay and not being completely blindsided by this behaviour. I told her I realized what was happening and that I was keeping my eyes and ears open as I recognized the start of bullying behaviour, and I wasn't about to take it again.

The idol comments, then the eye rolling as she had just talked to me then walked away, and then overloading my specific area in emerge when she was charge it was a continual pattern for about a year. It was the little things she did to make you feel 2 inches tall and therefore making her feel like big man on campus. Clearly, I was deemed a threat in her eyes and at that point I was able to have an opinion and voice it, when need be, regarding the care of my patients. There was also the point that she used to be on the IV team and was someone that other nurses went to for hard IV starts. I had started quickly to be someone who the newer nurses would come to, to try an IV after they hadn't been able to get it. Looking back this was also potentially an issue as people would start to come to me before they would go to her (as they may have assumed as she was charge, she was busy with charge things). It was less than a year before the constant comments and passive aggressive behaviour became a bit too much and I looked for work elsewhere.

It wasn't until I had already accepted a job at an adult emergency and was leaving that her behaviour became subtly more and more intolerable,

22 | BULLY ENCOUNTER #2

that I confronted her. It took me six weeks after I had already *left* the department and would pick up the occasional shift for me to finally say something to her.

I will say that did I didn't confront her at the most opportune time or in the best way. I happened to only see her as we were changing shifts and she was about to take an admitted patient upstairs. I quickly blurted out that her behaviour towards me over the last year was totally unacceptable and I wondered if everything was okay at home as usually someone who behaves this way could be trying to reach out for help. She seemed shocked, but I was already over it at that point, so I left and went home. I continued to pick up the occasional shift there and sure enough the next shift I picked up she was there, and wouldn't you know that she was the charge nurse that day as well.

I cringed looking up at the white board and seeing her name there. There was no way I was going to be able to get through twelve hours without seeing her or talking to her with where and I were placed in the department. I decided to keep my chin up and just hold the line. I'd said my peace and I could move on but knowing bullies as I do, I'm sure that she was going to have something to say about it. Whether or not it would be to my face would be another story.

Before I even could turn around the hair on the back of my neck prickled and I knew she was behind me. It wasn't more than a beat that passed by before she asked if we could have a talk. We walked into one of the empty trauma rooms and closed the doors. My heart *pounding* in my chest and my hands starting to shake. I knew that this probably wasn't going to go well but I had said something, and this was her opportunity to say her peace in return. It was the least I could do...I guess, the anger at being bullied still roiling in my gut.

We had a very adult and open conversation about how the previous conversation went and I did apologize for doing it at shift change, but that had been the first time I had seen her since I left for the other ER. I told her I was going to let it go until she made a snide comment at my expense. "For the last time" I thought as I had approached her at that time. She stated that I had blindsided her at shift change and right before she was about to take a patient upstairs to be admitted. She told me that she had no idea how I felt. She spoke about how after she had taken the patient upstairs, she had cried in the resus room. She confessed to me the part where I asked if something was wrong at home was what had bothered her the most. I told her I was just trying to make sense of her behaviour. I can't remember if we hugged it out or not, but I cried. I usually do with confrontation. I can't remember if she cried but either way, we called a truce. The rest of the shift seemingly went by without incident. I tried to purposefully ask if she needed any help with anything and tried to be as polite as I could be. It's hard to unpack a year's worth of behaviour and letting those emotions seemingly fester. It's even harder to then try and turn your reactions around and let the resentment and hurt go.

It still felt horribly awkward anytime we worked together after that, but at least she stayed out of my hair. It wasn't too long before that ER had enough part time staff and I stopped getting calls to come in. It was the first time I had stood up for myself and as extraordinarily anxiety producing as it was, it was gratifying to know I broke through her shell and made her think about her actions and how she spoke to people. Things may also have improved as I had already left the department and was working that ER *very* causally to cover sick calls. It was way easier to confront her at this time as I had already left the department and had nothing left to lose.

I still within my current job need to visit that ER occasionally to drop off a patient and I always wonder if I'll see her. The best part? I could care *less* about it. I said my peace and now I'm moving on.

23 | BULLY ENCOUNTER #3

I KEPT looking for the perfect ER fit. My new position had a big learning curve. This ER was the crème de la crème and one I'd never dreamt that I'd be working at. In this ER, patients were being sent to us from elsewhere. The acuity, reputation and the traumas were the things I was most looking forward to. It was a fast fit, and I was so happy about it.

I quickly moved through the ranks and was being prepped to move into trauma training within six months of being there—an accomplishment that I was so freaking excited for. I was on cloud nine! Trauma was the thing that I had loved most in all the other hospitals, but at this location the patients came to us. The number of times I had dropped patients off at this ER during my time working in Southern Ontario were too many to count. I was always blown away by the sheer number of people who would be there when I came alone with my one patient and was so excited to finally be on the opposite end of it. The bonus was that my previous experience in other ER's meant that I would occasionally get to see friends pass through as they were transferring a patient. It was great. The team nursing model was a little difficult to get used to in comparison to just being responsible for my set four or five patients in the other ER's, but it worked out well. Everything was going fine until the day I crossed paths with my third bully, another charge nurse. There were only two instances with this person, but it was enough for to again start looking for another job.

The first incident happened when this charge nurse and I were working in a room with up to ten patients (three of whom could be in the hallway). One patient had been there all night and the report we got from nightshift was that she was waiting for a consult from medicine. They said that medicine had originally seen her and deferred her for a surgical consult who she'd seen during the night. Now she was deferred *back* to medicine. It had been a few hours since the surgery resident had seen the patient and nightshift was waiting for medicine to reassess and write admission orders.

In our charting system we have a tracker that is a board of all the patient names. It electronically keeps track of how long the patient has been there, who is most responsible physician (MRP), where in the ER process that patient is (awaiting to be seen, waiting for labs, waiting for diagnostics, waiting consult, admission status and discharge status). Within all those process interventions there is a timer to see how long we've waited for something. This allows us, at a quick glance, to know how long it's been since imaging or since a consult has been called, accepted, arrived, and then admitted.

On this day, the problem was that the poor patient was punted from medicine to surgery back and forth *several* times. With it being team nursing I couldn't keep track of what service we were waiting on to see the patient so I would change the tracker to whatever service we were waiting for this caused the timer to restart each time we were waiting for that service. This was a problem for the charge nurse. She didn't realize what was happening so while the tracker *looked* like only an hour or two since the consult was called, the patient had actually been in the department for over thirty-six hours. When she asked me what had happened, I explained the situation and she yelled at me in front of six patients (including the patient who was in the middle of this) and their family members. She yelled that it was unsafe for the patient, how I'd messed up the tracker every time I changed it, and how the patient's lack of admission orders meant the other nurses wouldn't know how to take care of her.

It was shocking. I'd been there maybe nine months; this was not an acute care area but a kind of holding area for those who needed stretchers but not necessarily cardiac monitoring. I tried to tell her we were still in keeping with emergency documentation standard and doing vitals every four hours, but she was having *none* of it. After the yelling incident, she went back into her charge area and didn't speak to me for the rest of the day (which in a department of over fifteen or sixteen Registered Nurses was not uncommon). However, I was *done* with being someone's punching bag. I was mortified that she had yelled at me and then horrified that she'd done it in front of all my patients.

So, I emailed my manager describing what had happened. I didn't delay. About a month went by before my manager got back to me in a face-to-

23 | BULLY ENCOUNTER #3

face meeting, (oddly in the same room that the incident had taken place). She asked what I wanted to do about my email. I hadn't worked with that person since it happened as I was part time and she was full time. I knew the charge nurse was new to the role and I couldn't imagine managing a department with upwards of forty-two patients. I hoped it was a one-off situation and indicated that I'd give her the benefit of the doubt and let it go. My manager agreed and walked away.

It wasn't even half the shift later when *it happened again.* The same freaking day I choose to let it go, she yells at me *a second time* in front of a room full of patients and their families. I was shocked and couldn't say a word. I was so mad at myself for not saying anything when she was in my face for a second time. I was still standing in a little corner cubicle that was the nursing station when she came back. I decided it was time to say something.

"Can I talk to you for a minute?" I asked moving us further into the corner of the cubicle to get some privacy, even though she'd not given me the same courtesy. I didn't want my patients to hear anything of what I was about to say to her.

"What?" She asked pointedly.

"I wanted to say that it's unprofessional for you to yell at me in front of my patients. This is the second time that it's happened and I'm not about to take it." I said quietly, my entire insides shaking as I found the courage to finally say something.

"*What?*" she asked again, raising her voice.

I repeated myself. "It's unprofessional to yell at me in front of my patients and you will not do it again." I said it a little more firmly but still quietly enough that I hoped my patients didn't hear.

"If that's your main concern, then you're in the wrong profession," she snapped and walked away.

I let out a deep breath that I didn't know I was holding. I tried to collect myself, as it was still early in the morning of this dayshift and my partner had been on break as it all went down. When she came back, I explained what'd happened and the saddest part was that my co-worker wasn't at all surprised by this behavior.

"Oh, that's just her," she said.

"That's not a reason," I said through gritted teeth, the anger starting to settle in.

I emailed my manager, updating her on what had happened. I asked for a meeting to resolve it, as it was completely unprofessional and I was *done*. Later that same day we have the meeting. I say my peace and recount what happened. Then it was the charge nurse's turn to explain her behaviour. She brought up the fact that a few months previously I'd asked for a shift change that she had accepted. The day before the shift, she learned that I'd done a last-minute swap with someone and hadn't let her know. I said I was sorry and explained that, at the time, I was doing many shift swaps as I was routinely double-booked between my two jobs. Neither one gave the option of submitting availability. I didn't remember the incident but apologized regardless.

"It's unacceptable. I was about to make daycare changes and drive an hour to come in—and you just say you're sorry?" She pointedly askes.

"Yes, I'm sorry about the switch, but that was months ago and it doesn't give you the right to yell at me in front of my patients and their families...twice" I say firmly.

"I was just worried about the patient in the hallway that you left alone." She spits out. "How could you leave him to be the last one assessed? Where's your nursing judgement?" she asks, her voice starting to rise.

"The report that I received was that he was the most stable of our ten patients and the plan was for physiotherapy to see him before he was discharged—so yes, he was the last to be seen," I reply.

"Well, I watched him all morning. He was falling out of the bed and having trouble breathing. There were no vitals charted and it's already ten am," she hissed.

"Again," I said, "he was the most stable and going home so I focussed on the patients who I thought were sicker," I stated.

"Everybody needed to be seen by eight with vitals done. If you can't hack it in this emerge then maybe you shouldn't work here," she quipped, a devious half-smile on her lips.

She had a point. I did leave the patient to be assessed last as I assumed that the nightshift report was correct. It turned out that the patient's oxygen saturations were about 88% and he *was* having trouble breathing.

23 | BULLY ENCOUNTER #3

We moved him into our room to see if we could figure out what was going on, but he ended up on a continuous positive airway pressure (CPAP) mask in *her* area by the time the meeting took place in the afternoon. It was a mistake on my end. I took full responsibility, as I wasn't about to blame my team nursing partner that day. I was the one with more experience in emergency and should've known better.

The meeting went around and around, and really progressing forward. I worried my partner was getting inundated with orders and drowning with the workflow. I asked to leave the meeting and return to work.

I was so frustrated. What started out as a bullying meeting got turned around into an issue with my practice, and the bullying complaint fell to the wayside. I remember telling my partner that this was *exactly* why bullying isn't reported. It gets turned around because management doesn't want to deal with the more complicated bullying issue. My solution was to look for full-time work instead of the two part-time jobs I had. I got the *hell* out — moving to the first ER I could find.

The saddest part is that I think I could've been happy there. The pace was amazing, the medicine being practiced was above and beyond what I'd ever seen before. One time there was a code blue called and as I was charting, the doctor cracked the guy's chest open and started performing *internal cardiac massage*. The doctor literally had his hands in this guy's chest massaging the heart. It was so routine for them that no one was like, "hey look over here." (Side note: coolest procedure I've ever seen.)

I was so close to being trauma trained that I could taste it but this bully usually worked trauma and the thought of having to team nurse with her was the least appealing thing I could think of at that time. So, I moved on...again. This was the third job I had left specifically due to bullying. Ironically, I'm only making this connection as *I'm writing this*. How could I have missed that this was the reason I kept moving?

Thirteen years. It took me thirteen years to put this together.

At least now I will have a reply when asked why I keep changing jobs. My friends have joked for years that they can't keep up with where I'm working. I just took it in stride because I was moving around a lot. Bullying. Bullying is the reason I moved around so much.

THE MORAL OF THESE STORIES

The easy take away is that I run away when faced with bullying. Over the years, and in retelling the stories, I can see that I've grown to the point where at least I'm speaking up for myself and at least I'm taking responsibility for my actions. Sometimes I say things and I do things that, if taken out of context, may also be considered bullying. You better believe that I am so self-aware of what I say, how I say it, and how it may be interpreted because I don't ever want anyone to feel the way I've felt. Sometimes personalities don't mesh. If I'm stressed, I may say something in haste. Sometimes I get overwhelmed and I expect people to work a certain way without asking them. It's all in how you communicate. We know that 90% of communication is nonverbal. Take a minute to analyze yourself and your behaviour. If you've said or done something that you feel guilty about, just say sorry. You have no idea how much an apology would have changed things for me. You never know what someone is dealing with at home. You don't want your behaviour to be the thing that tips them over the edge.

Here are some responses to various instances of bullying that are starting to be taught in second year of nursing school. *Second year.* Bullying is so pervasive; it's time they focused on it in school. Maybe in thirty years we'll be better off for it. Think of this tool as a cheat sheet—appropriate responses for uncomfortable situations.[1]

- Verbal affront (covert or overt snide remarks). *What do you mean by that comment?*
- Non-verbal innuendo (raising of eyebrows, making faces). *I see from your facial expression that you might be confused. What else do you need to know?*
- With-holding information (related to one's practice or a patient). *I feel that you aren't telling me everything I need to know.*
- Sabotage (interference in production, work). *I feel this should not have happened. We need to talk about this privately.*
- Undermining activities (to weaken, injure, destroy by secret or

23 | BULLY ENCOUNTER #3

insidious means). *I feel that you don't trust me. Will you tell me why?*

- Infighting (bickering with peers). *We need to stop this behavior and learn to work together.*
- Backstabbing (betraying a friend or an associate). *I don't feel comfortable talking about (person's name) when they are not present.*
- Broken confidences. *This is information that should remain confidential.*
- Scapegoating (assigning the blame to one person for the shortcomings of others). *We can't blame one person for everything that goes wrong.*
- Gossiping (idle talk, groundless rumor). *This is inappropriate conversation that should not be taking place.*

I know that it takes internal fortitude to confront someone, but the satisfaction that comes when you stand up for yourself is more than worth it. To have your say and walk away without escalating the situation is a talent. If you're not ready to tackle face-to-face conversations, start keeping a journal regarding circumstances, behaviours, your response, their response, and aggravating factors. It might give you a better understanding of the situation and if nothing else, it gives you backup if you decide to confront the person or involve your manager. In nursing you know—if it's not charted it's not done.

If you're not keeping tabs on bullying behaviours, including witnesses, it potentially could be swept under the carpet. We know there are managers who don't want to rock the boat. They will be the ones who ask so many questions that you may start to doubt what happened. This is a poor managerial style that may cause you so much aggravation that you put up your hands and say forget it. But don't do it! Knowing your employers code of conduct is key to raising concerns. If you get nowhere with your own manager there is always the option of escalating the complaint to your manager's boss, taking it up the chain of command until something is done. A lot of employers will promote that they have a zero-tolerance policy for bullying and yet when it is brought to their attention nothing gets done. Filing a complaint may make your life harder on a day-to-day basis, but if that person's behaviour escalates or they retaliate you can again take action. A journal with support this and provide evidence to your employer of your concerns.

If I'd kept a journal with all the various encounters with bullies that I've had over my thirteen-year career span, she' be a hefty book. Telling my stories would've been helped by having more examples to demonstrate if there was a pattern to the offensive behaviour. Also, if you have a safety occurrence or incident report that you are supposed to fill out when bullying happens, please fill do that too. This goes double for physical altercations.

No one should ever have to stress about coming into work.

23 | BULLY ENCOUNTER #3

JOURNAL PROMPTS

Have you ever been in a situation similar to what I've described?
_____
_____
_____
_____

What happened?
_____
_____
_____
_____

How did you handle it?
_____
_____
_____
_____

24 | SHOWING UP TO A NEW UNIT

WITH ALL THIS TALK of me moving from unit to unit, I thought it would be a good idea to include "tips and tricks" on how to join a new unit quickly and effectively. I often joke that when I arrive to a new unit my first questions are:

- where to put my stuff?
- where to put my food?
- where the medication dispenser is?
- where the bathrooms are?

and most importantly,

- where we cry.

The truth is that many units are designed the same way, and it's usually just about figuring out where things are. The answer is to make friends with the word clerk, the personal support workers, and the environmental aids (aka housekeeping). These people are the heart and soul of a unit and are potentially less likely to move around as much as nurses do. They know the ins and outs of the unit, they know who does what, and they know the entire history of the unit (aka the gossip).

Knowing the gossip in a new unit can help you figure out the people a little bit faster: who likes working where, who doesn't get along, who is part of a clique and who likes to gossip? Knowing the personalities of your co-workers is a huge deal. If I've ever had concerns about a nurse I was working with (e.g., were they trustworthy?), I casually talk to the healthcare aides and very politely bring up that person to see if they volunteered any information. Thankfully they almost always do. This is another instance of trusting your gut. If you're working with someone and are not getting great vibes, chances are that's who that person is. As always, if somebody flat out shows you who they are and that they are not a nice person, trust that too.

If you were not comfortable of being on the floor within a few months, you can also just keep quiet and stay in the background. In the first few months, people trying to figure you out too. It gives you some time to figure things out. Some of the best insights have come while charting, but keeping my ears open at the same time. People talk. Listen to what they say. Watch how they interact with patients, other nurses and support staff. If someone is nice to you because you're the nurse and then completely awful to the support staff, you might want to watch your back.

The sooner you figure out new routines and processes, the better your life is going to be. Every unit (regardless of type) has their own quirks and ways to do things. It's hard to learn new ways of doing things but sometimes it's just easier to do it their way while they get used to you. After some time use your own judgement regarding the effectiveness of the methods being used. If the work gets done, and gets done safely, usually that's enough.

Other quick tips

- Figure out if the charge nurse has a specific chair in the department. Do not sit in that spot. You'll thank me later.

- Try not to say, "but at my old unit we did it this way." I know everybody has their own experiences, judgement, and knowledge but if you're *that* person who is vocally comparing the new unit to the old unit, people are going to stop talking to you.

- Be helpful to the other nurses when starting a new unit. If your work is done, please offer to help others. You never know when you're going to be dealt a crap assignment. Having co-workers to cover your back is always a good thing. This won't happen if you don't make the first move. No one will save you.

- Do what you can, when you can and only take a break once most of the work is done. This is especially true in the ER. Don't put off doing vitals, an assessment, a med pass—do it all at the same time. You never know what's going to come through the door and completely mess up your day. If you get everybody fluffed and puffed early, then at least your patients have seen you and you

24 | SHOWING UP TO A NEW UNIT

will have an idea about how sick your patients are. If you have a task, and there's no time constraint, don't put it off. If they want am labs that means you can do them at four in the morning if you have time. Don't wait until six am to draw labs because that leaves a potentially critical result arriving at a time that puts dayshift already behind.

- If you have a minute, give everybody a warm blanket. Seriously. It's just going to make your day easier so offer them the damn blanket.
- Figure out everybody's cliques early and see if you want to be in them or not. If you prefer days or night shifts, then see if anyone will volunteer the information about who wants the opposite shift and if you can swap with them.

The simple answer of what will make your easier when it comes to swapping units, is to sit back and watch the action. Note how people interact with each other, how the doctors talk to the nurses, and how problems are dealt with.

You'll end up with answers to questions you never even thought to ask.

JOURNAL PROMPTS

Do you have any favorite new routines when starting a new unit?
___
___
___
___

What aspect of starting a new unit scares or intimidates you?
___
___
___
___

25 | A NOTE ABOUT COVID-19

IF YOU ARE NEWER to nursing or are in nursing school, I would like to formally apologize for any wrongdoings by anyone who has currently been in the medical field over the last couple of years. This is not us. This is not the medicine that I've known throughout my career. We are all *not okay* and sadly the residual burnout, exhaustion, fear and worry may be coloring how we react to situations and people. We're not the easy going, funny and goofy selves we normally are. We are tired, scared and overworked to the point of caregiver fatigue and compassion fatigue. The amount of moral and ethical dilemmas that many of us have faced has pushed us passed our limits.

Work used to be fun and so were our co-workers. Depending on the unit, we would have potlucks every Sunday night, go out for wine tours and hang out with each other. Our Christmas parties would be paired with EMS, and they were *legendary*. Not these last years though. COVID segregated us from friends and family, pushed us to handle childcare while still being expected to work full-time hours during a global pandemic. We finally got recognition for the hard work we've always done, but it took us putting our lives and the lives of our families on the line to get it. Receiving thanks from our communities was validating and yet so at odds with how we are normally treated (in the ER anyways). I have always likened working the ER to being in an abusive relationship with the public. You love to help, but you get treated badly every single day. You don't realize just how much you've endured only *halfway* through your career until you sit down and start to recount story after story—trauma after trauma.

Going through COVID has given me a *much* better understanding of why people who survived going to war, simply *never* talked about it again. It's too painful to keep rehashing those memories and especially with that generation, going to therapy wasn't an option. How thankful

I am that things have changed, but I understand. I understand why the trauma and horrors witnessed were never spoken of again. There were many types of stress experienced by most (if not all) medical practitioners during COVID. These stressors included the constant fear of contracting COVID-19 and then infecting others because of inadequate supplies of PPE. These were the mental hurdles we had to navigate everyday just to be able to show up to work.

To delve into those emotions and makes sense of what we were feeling, and how we felt our worlds were crumbling around us is beyond most of us. I've never been so close to a mental breakdown as I was during the first and second waves of COVID. To be honest, if I had to sit down and truly relive moments of COVID and the fear, I think I would be swallowed whole by my emotions and fears. Being face-to-face with your own mortality is not fun.

I used to think I had a healthy perspective on death and dying. COVID showed me just how unprepared I was for thoughts of leaving my children without a mother and the related emotions that would pop up at the least opportune times. How did we manage such feelings? We shoved them down. Deep. Feelings of fear, worry, anxiety, stress, and angst were locked up. It was easier to pretend that everything was going to be fine than being real about just how frightened and worried we truly were.

Ironically, we all showed up to work and no one called in sick. Why? We were saving our sick days for when we assumed we would eventually get sick. It was not a question of *if* we would get sick, but *when*. In the early days before the first lockdown, we all (kind of) laughed it off like it was no worse than the flu. Then the mask mandates, the policy changes and the rates of people coming into the ER plummeted. It was the weirdest feeling sitting there watching Wuhan fall, then Italy. Pictures from New York with people wearing garbage bags for personal protective equipment. Then it came to Ontario. Thankfully COVID barely grazed us the first wave, but in the moment, it felt like the bottom of my world could drop out at any moment. With school and daycares closed, we had no access to childcare; my parents were unable to help us due to both my husband and I being frontline workers and high risk.

I did what I could. I changed my schedule to work straight nights,

25 | A NOTE ABOUT COVID-19

came home, watched the kids. My husband would be home around four pm, I would try and get an hour nap before going back into work. The stress and worry of contracting COVID and exposing my family were my biggest concerns and living nightmare. To say that March to June 2020 were the darkest days and nights of my life is not an overstatement. I was a wreck. I would overeat one minute and then not be hungry for the rest of the day. I wasn't sleeping and could feel myself drift away from those I loved. It was the beginning of the worst episode of depression and despair that I've ever experienced.

And then...the light.

Some of the local university's students had started a support program for frontline workers. It was a fluke that I even saw the flyer. There were students willing to come into my home to watch my kids while I slept so I applied. This program saved the small fragment of sanity I had left. I would come home at around 8:00 am, after a nightshift, and at 9:00 am one of our two designated volunteers showed up. These were two of the sweetest souls I have ever encountered, and they saved me. *Saved me.* One was a nursing student in her last year and the other was in his last year of teachers' college. They are, and always will be, saints in my book. They gave me hope that there was still some good in the world and that people would rally together to support each other in whatever way was necessary to keep things moving.

While the volunteering program officially ended in April, both of my volunteers were willing to stay on with me as daycares were still not open in June. One volunteer finally let me pay her, while the other continued to refuse to take my money. My faith in humanity had been restored.

In a cruel twist of fate, just as I had started to feel the edges of moral fatigue and compassion fatigue receding, a critical incident with a co-worker pushed me over the edge into full-fledged burnout.

26 | THE FINAL STRAW

IT WAS THE MIDDLE of May and while we were still in lockdown, ER visits had decreased from seeing 60-70 people a day down to 15-20 people. We were finally fully staffed (if not overstaffed) due to the closure of the OR. My best friend and I were talking at her desk, and we witnessed a known toxic co-worker getting ready to go into a COVID isolation room about fifteen feet in front of us. The patient was one of the sickest we had seen in a long time and had a very high likelihood of COVID-19. We watched our colleague don her PPE, get all the things she needed ready and go into the room. The two of us continued to talk for a few minutes before we saw her exit the room. She didn't take off her PPE as she was supposed to. Instead, she went into an IV cart full of supplies, rifling around for a minute before heading back into the room.

We were gobsmacked. What did we just see? A level of fear rose so quickly in me that it was all I could do to *not* put on gloves and throw out the contents of the entire cart. I figured it was a mistake—she had just forgotten to take off the PPE in her haste to get what she needed. I was frozen in place for several minutes. I had no words as my throat was constricted by fear. I thought, if she had done this once, who knows what else she may have touched? We thought that we were all being diligent at keeping those isolated in the ER in the proper area— that we all had been following precautions to a tee. The thought of this trust being broken shattered me. I could no longer trust that the ER was "clean".

I let the charge nurse know that there'd been a breach in the cleanliness of the department and that something needed to be done. I eventually convinced her that the whole cart needed to be tossed, wiped down and restocked because we had no idea of what she touched and if anything had been contaminated. The charge said that the patient in question wasn't doing well and would need to be transferred out, so it would be taken care of as soon as possible. The patient was sent to another hospital within thirty to forty-five minutes. In that time the charge nurse tossed the entire cart. When the toxic co-worker returned from that transfer, she saw the charge nurse cleaning the cart. She asked what happened and was directed to talk to me.

"Hey, can I talk to you?" she demanded.

"Sure, actually I was meaning to talk to you too," I said.

We went into the empty resuscitation room. It's was early morning and thankfully there wasn't a lot happening in the department.

"Why did you have everything on the IV cart thrown out?" Another demand.

"Well, you came out of the isolation room with all of your PPE on and went through the cart. We didn't know what you had touched and what you hadn't. That patient was a high risk of being a positive COVID patient." I gently tried to get the point across that she had been in the wrong. "I get that sometimes we forget that we can't just go in and out of the rooms anymore due to COVID, but we can't risk spreading germs.".

"Well, I saw you and Christina there and I yelled at you for help."

"I'm sorry but I didn't hear you." I stayed calm, knowing this co-worker had a history of blowing up and becoming aggressive with confrontation.

"Look, I know I can be loud, and I know you heard me!" She argues, waving her arms for emphasis.

"No, I'm sorry but I *didn't* hear you. We both saw you going into the cart and then go back into the room." I say, still keeping my composure.

"Well, I did it on purpose because I saw both of you were watching." She says crossing her arms and standing straighter.

"What?" I squeak out, hoping like hell I'd misheard her.

"Yeah, I did it on purpose because I yelled to you guys, and nobody did anything, so I just grabbed it myself." She replies.

I couldn't believe what I was hearing. In the middle of a global pandemic when we're all struggling to keep our heads above water, she decided to do this. It was unfathomable. It was crazy. What kind person would purposefully put the entire department and their families at risk just to prove a point? At this point I stopped listening to what she was saying until she asked me questions about "the statistics." I had a niggling feeling that she maybe thought COVID wasn't as serious as it was being portrayed as in the media. I asked her where she got her information from.

26 | THE FINAL STRAW

"WHO (World Health Organization)" she said. OK I thought, that's a reputable source. Then she said that she liked to keep a finger on the world's news.

"So, what other news outlets do you use?" I asked.

"Well, I like to keep an eye on the States, I watch a lot of FOX news." She proudly states.

Oh my God.

She let me know that Georgia was opening its beaches that weekend and that she thought it was a great idea. She was also the co-worker who (to this day) doesn't wear her mask properly. I mentally *lost it*. To me, the department was effectively contaminated. There was no safe space to eat because who knows where or what she touched. I applied out and got a job in Post Anesthetic Care Room (PACU) or Recovery Room which continues to be one of the most sheltered and protected areas of the hospital system. Everyone coming through the door except for true surgical emergencies is swabbed for COVID, done and resulted.

The worst part was that I reported the malicious intent to my manager and was asked to let it go. It was bad enough to have a co-worker I didn't trust, let alone a manager who would let that kind of thing happen.

Of all the stories that I will talk about after COVID is done, this is the one I'll still be able to recount on my deathbed. The trauma was so multi-dimensional that it's taken several attempts to write it down. I continue to wonder just how badly COVID will impact me in five, ten or even twenty years from now. I wonder about the wounds that have been created but not understood. I wonder if I will ever be "normal" again or whether the pain and torment of the past two years will continually run in the background of my mind. I'd like to think I'll get to a point where I can go away on a vacation and not be worrying about my traumas peeking through at unexpected moments.

I'd love nothing more than to be in a shaded, comfy hammock by the water with the wind rocking me gently and to have nothing but peaceful thoughts. If nothing else, it's a goal to work towards.

EXERCISE: UNPACKING THE EFFECTS OF THE PANDEMIC

It's time to take stock of how you're feeling post-COVID. Take a minute to breathe as this may bring up *a lot* of emotions. Take your time. Be gentle with yourself. Write whatever you can. Let it all out. If nothing else this may be useful in the future, to be able to look back at how it started vs. how it's going in 15-20 years. Let this be a safe space to let out your deepest fears and worries.

How has COVID-19 affected you?
_____
_____
_____
_____

What have been the biggest hurdles you have had to overcome?
_____
_____
_____
_____

What was the most confusing part of your experience?
_____
_____
_____
_____

Were there any silver linings?
_____
_____
_____
_____

27 | HOW TO SURVIVE NIGHTSHIFTS

AHH NIGHTSHIFTS, they're either the bane of a nurse's existence or a much-anticipated reprise from day shift craziness. There will always be pros and cons for each shift and depending on the life stage you're in, a shift that used to work for you may have changed and you'd prefer something different.

Nightshifts are mysterious to people who've never worked them. They can't seem to wrap their heads around having to stay up all night and then try and sleep during the day....and it shows! People who cut their grass and build stuff in their backyards at 8 am in the morning drive me insane. As someone who, for at least ¾ of my career has been in nightshift, these types of people are the worst. It's also not helpful when these same people can't understand why you're sleeping at five pm (if you're *lucky*). I find the easiest way to explain it is to tell them to switch the time from pm to am.

It's not rocket science. Calling me at two pm may seem reasonable. *However,* I just got off nights and am going back again so you're calling me at (my) two am. How would they feel if I called them at two am? They probably wouldn't be super excited about it. Sometimes I dream of doing this to friends or family members that repeatedly forget my schedule. I have (maybe on one or two occasions) called a friend's cellphone at three am while at work and leave a voicemail:

"Hey what's up, I was just driving around and wondered if you wanted to get a coffee, I mean it's my two pm so that means you're up, right? Call me back!"

I can be a little vindictive if seriously pissed off enough with someone's behavior.

There has only been one person who has been consistently mindful of my schedule: my dad. My dad used to work shiftwork, so he *gets it*. If he calls at two pm and I happen to answer because I forgot to turn my ringer off and I sound tired...he asks me if I just got off work. If I say yes, he says to get back to bed and *hangs up on me*. I laugh because it would seem to be such a rude gesture, but he doesn't want me waking up and if he hangs up, I have no other option than to go back to bed. I love that man *so much* it hurts. No matter what I'm doing, it seems like he's done it before and is there when I stumble. He used to tell me how best to get ready for nightshift: Sleep when you can before the first shift. Learn to nap wherever you are—also fantastic advice. Over the years I have developed a nightshift routines/ritual.

PREP FOR NIGHTSHIFT 1

Have a nap before the first nightshift. An hour, three hours—it doesn't matter, as long as you get a nap. You never know when you'll get a shift where you get no sleep for twelve plus hours and it's those days that you'll wish you'd laid down when you had a chance. Blackout curtains should be one of your first purchases, whether you're in school or graduated.

After the nap. Treat it like you're getting up and ready for work. Flip into your morning routine. Shower, get dressed, hair, make up (I know, it's a joke to put on makeup for nights but sometimes I just want to look pretty). Have a cup of coffee or tea. Sit and read and have a quiet moment if you can before the chaos of nights.

Compression stockings: If you can get fitted for compression stockings, I *highly* suggest them. Nothing is worse than running around for twelve hours and having your feet ache for thirty minutes when you get home. Many benefit programs cover compression stockings with a doctor's note. Also, orthotics were the best decision I ever made when I realized how much my feet ached after a busy shift.

Prep light meals. I like to pack one heavy meal for "dinner" and then a lighter meal/snack for closer to the end of shift. Also, just always have easy on-the-run snacks available. If you're unit happens to get "relaxed" enough, (I'm not saying the Q-word) bring an activity that is easily picked up and put down. A book, word puzzle, sudoku, cross stitching etc.

27 | HOW TO SURVIVE NIGHTSHIFTS

GETTING READY FOR ANOTHER NIGHTSHIFT

Once you're home and going to be returning for another nightshift, eat something of substance that will hold you over for a few hours, perform bedtime routines and then get into that bed asap. That's it. It's the easiest way to swap into nights.

Sleep as late as you can (four or five pm preferably). Then, when you get up, treat it like your morning. It's hard to get the hang of it at first, but with time it gets easier. Doing things like making sure you eat and pee before going to bed, have the room be a bit cool, use blackout curtains and make sure to turn your phone and smart watch onto silent with all vibrations off will tee you up for success.

COMING OFF YOUR LAST NIGHT SHIFT FOR A SET

The idea is still the same. Get ready for bed asap, eat and pee before going to bed. If you normally take medications to help with sleep maybe avoid them after the last shift. Try and get up around 2-3 pm to give yourself a "wake window" before going to bed later that evening. Take medications at your regular bedtime after your last shift to help promote you getting back into "dayshift mode."

JOURNAL PROMPTS

What are your nightshift rituals? Do you have a schedule you like to follow?
_____
_____

What helps you fall asleep and stay asleep?
_____
_____

What's one thing you could do to make your sleep habits work better for you?
_____
_____

28 | WILL

SOMETIMES WHEN you meet someone new, you rush to conclusions about them. It's not your fault. You've learned to trust your gut and you go with the flow. After a year of knowing Will, (and being someone who generally is good at reading people) I was completely surprised by his transformation since returning to my current ER. Will was a nurse for four years who decided to switch to become a paramedic and then changed again—returning to being an ER nurse. He's an older gentleman who is a soft spoken, funny and easy-going guy. He never gets worked up about anything. The department could be burning down around him, and he'd still act like everything was going to be okay.

Will and I had worked together for a year on and off and got along well. There were plenty of conversations around nursing and EMS and how things have changed. One day the topic turned to ghost stories. If you've worked in nursing for any length of time you know that ghost stories, often come up on nightshift. During breaks talks will turn to whether anyone has heard, seen, or felt anything or work.

Everyone has a story or two. It may not be from their current department, but almost all the nurses I know have either a story of their own or one they've heard someone else tell. (E.g., cardiac monitors in resuscitation rooms suddenly turning on and showing an accurate cardiac rhythm but not actually being attached to anything. People laying down for a break and hearing their name, or voices call out. The feeling of being squeezed tight or thinking that you've seen something out of the corner of your eye are just a few of my own ghost stories and those of co-workers.)

This was one of those nights where we were able to sit around the nursing station and talk with each other. Someone brought up ghost stories and I shared my thoughts and experiences. Then Will shared his. It turns out his extended family had been part of a famous haunting in the 1980's—so famous that the local police had even been involved at the time. It had left a profound and lasting mark on Will. He grew up with this story being told and re-told by various family members. He explained how he flat out refused to give into the thoughts of ghosts (or anything along that line) as it gave too much power to the fear that was an almost constant presence in his psyche.

I decided to share my quirky views on spirit, including my death rituals and other experiences that I've had. This includes how I always talk to myself, asking any spirit listening to not to bother me when I'm trying to have my break on nightshift. It sounds odd, I know. I believe there may be more to life than what I can see with my eyes and it gives me comfort to think that someone may be watching my back, spiritually speaking. It's one way I've come to terms the hurt and pain I see on a daily basis.

I explained this to Will. I asked, what was the harm in talking to a spirit and letting them know that you know they're there but not in a place to acknowledge them any more than that. A lightbulb went off in Will's eyes. He had been in fear for so long, that the negative energy of the previous haunting would follow him. For decades he'd worried about every bump in the night. When his sons would say that they saw things in the night, (as kids do) he was terrified. He worried for years about what could happen, when it could happen, and if it was going to happen to him.

After this conversation, Will started talking to spirits. He began by acknowledge spirits but let them know that he wasn't ready to hear anything or see anything from them and he was not ready to do anything more than just a acknowledge their presence. He and I starting talking more about what I have seen, felt and sensed through the years and the same for him. He asked about my crystals, what they were for and what they did. Did I think they helped? (Which, of course I did). I asked if it even mattered if I thought that the crystals brought good "juju" into the department and did it matter if he *didn't*.

If my beliefs keep me calm and helps me get organized (and potentially protects the department from bad things happening!) why not utilize it? Will was intrigued. Now, Will is someone who loves to research the hell out of a new hobby and his interest in crystals was no different. We'd discuss the crystals I had and the crystals he was interested in. We discussed their properties, including were they simply nice to look at. Will began to buy crystals in bulk, starting with rose quartz and selenite. Crystals would appear each shift on my desk and he'd share his extra crystals with our co-workers on the same line. This was beyond kind of him. We started to refer to ourselves as the "crystal crew". What I find funny is that when I finally opened up about my interests and beliefs, people listened. Now we're all having a lot of fun talking about our crystals. The fact that I had misjudged my co-workers and thought that I was alone in my kooky beliefs was my mistake. I would've never in a thousand years thought Will would've been interested in crystals, and yet here we are.

I guess that's the part that floors me the most is that everybody has the capacity to change their mind, to go with the flow, accept new ideas and even run with them. It makes me so happy. A change of mindset meant that Will finally found comfort. He took charge of a situation he previously feared. It started with a tweak in thinking about ghosts, spirits, or a presence.

Months of conversations about crystals and spirits had gone by when Will remembered something. It was a memory hidden deep in the back of his mind—that his mother used to read tarot. She used a simple deck of cards (not actual tarot) and he remembered people coming to the house to look for answers from her. The moment he realized that his mom was into the spiritual side of things was a game changer. I asked if maybe it was his mom that was trying to get his attention, to make herself known.

He never thought that whatever was making bumps in the night could be someone who he loved dearly. Because of his family history he could only imagine a spirit with a negative connotation and that's what kept him stuck in a place of fear. His mind-set change boggles my brain because I used to be where he was—afraid of every sound that I heard. I used to worry about seeing or hearing "something" at work. Now when I go for break on a night shift I will either say out loud (or in my head), "I understand you're here, I understand you want to be acknowledged, but I'm just going for a break, so if you could not scare me that would be great." I understand how nuts I sound but I've never felt more at peace at work than I do now. I have a level of comfort working with the dead or those close to dying that I didn't before.

It's just so funny how one chance conversation and baring of one's soul on a regular ER night shift can change someone's life and perceptions so drastically. Will recently shared that he can see auras. "Can't you see the fuzzy line kind of surrounding everyone?" he asked.

I said, "No. I can't see that line."

He responds with, "Oh, I just thought everybody could see it." In this moment, Will realized he was special.

Watching someone who you've (kind of) mentored grow as a person, while already being an adult, is amazing. To witness someone, dive in headfirst with reckless abandon to embrace a new hobby warms my cold heart.

It makes me realize that we are all capable of change and growth regardless of what someone else may think.

29 | GHOST STORIES

MOST OF THE TIME a nightshift can just be as busy as dayshift. On the flipside, there are some ER night shifts where I wouldn't see a single patient. The eerie sensations and hearing every sound in an empty department is off-putting to say the least. If you want to start an interesting conversation with your coworkers, ask them about their ghost stories because I guarantee you're going to hear at least three or four.

I don't know if hospital ghost stories are prevalent because so many people pass through a hospital in a short time or because the rate of people dying in the building is high. You can go on Amazon right now and find books of nursing horror stories, nursing ghost stories, hospital horror stories and hospital paranormal experiences.

I have many ghost stories and most of them took place in a brand-new hospital on their paediatric floor. I don't know what it was about the paediatric floor that changed things for me, but it was where I kept seeing things out of the corner of my eye, down long dark hallways in the early mornings of night shift. This was also when I figured out that I was an empath and maybe that had something to do with what I was suddenly sensing.

One of my more vivid memories happened when I fell asleep while on break. I had a vivid dream that I was in the exact room where I was sleeping but playing on the floor next to me were two little boys who were roughly the same age as my own two children (who are a boy and a girl). There was something eerily similar between my kids and the two children in my dream. They felt real and seemed to be right in front of me. I remember waking myself and not having any idea whether the dream had actually happened. After that incident I was unable to rest in that room. I couldn't get the incident out of my head.

On that same paediatric floor there was also a family-style apartment in the back of the unit that you could take a break in. The apartment was originally designed for patients and their families if they had an extended stay on the unit, but thankfully almost all the children who we treated were in and back home within a few days. Again, while taking a break, I had a dream where I could have sworn, I was exactly where I was. I thought I heard someone talking about a glucose that had been done and that it was 5.4. I remember sitting up and saying "oh that's not too bad" before laying back down. To this day, I don't know if that was a dream or if I did actually sit up and speak out loud—either way it was a wake-up call.

After that, I decided that *something* more was going on. I wasn't vocal about it at first, but I certainly am now. I truly am laying out all my traumas, baring my soul and letting out all my kooky, woo-woo beliefs. If you meet me in person, (let alone work with me) I may talk about spirit or intuition. I definitely would share my interest in crystals. I'm 90% sure I'm going to say something that you probably weren't expecting me to say (which may also make my life a little bit more fun along the way).

Every day I become more confident in myself and my abilities and in my knowledge, skill and judgement. As a result, I am opening up and letting others in. My poor coworkers know this but when it's the same three or four people that I work with on the daily, I've got to be me!

Granted, I do filter myself to patients, as we all do, but I feel a level of freedom, openness and release that makes me wonder why I didn't do this sooner. Instead of fearing my empathetic nature, I've channeled it into being the best nurse that I can be. We all have the capability to be more empathetic and intuitive. Chances are you're more intuitive than you realize. The fact that I've come into my own during a time of unprecedented stress, worry, panic and fear makes me feel better, more hopeful and optimistic. I am also less afraid for a future that may have COVID or other illnesses in it. We all have a choice about whether we show up to work. I believe the ones who do, are the bravest people I know.

> *All we can do is build enough resilience to get through the challenges of our career and not be scarred by it for the rest of our lives.*

29 | GHOST STORIES

JOURNAL PROMPT

What's your ghost story?
___
___
___
___
___

30 | MY BEST STORY

OF COURSE, I am sharing my "best" story and my "most told story". Every nurse has them. The "best" story usually revolves around ghosts. This is that story.

It was early morning and I was working in the ER. We received a patch from EMS calling about a vital sign absent child (VSA). This is a few years after my first paediatric code, and I dreaded repeating it. Everyone started bustling around, getting ready for the incoming code blue. I asked if I could be the one who stays behind and cares for the rest of the department. Everyone agreed to the plan and I'm was more than a little relieved to sit the call out. Had I been needed, I willingly would have helped, but if there was an option to save myself a further trauma, I'd take it.

Five, six, seven minutes slowly tick by. Everyone surrounded the trauma bed with the smallest versions of the tools needed to save a young life. The silence spread as we gathered our thoughts and mentally ran through the various scenarios of what could happen and how to fix it.

The quiet is broken by the sound of ambulance sirens in the distance. You could feel tension bloom into the room as the sirens grew louder until they arrived right outside the ER doors. I took that as my cue to leave and check on the rest of the department. I let my charge nurse know that if she needed me or anything else to yell and I would be there in an instant.

As I walked away, I heard the glass doors to the ER ambulance bay slide open. The volume in the department was low as it was early in the morning, so the ER team slid the glass doors to the resus area, trying to contain the noise and retain as much confidentiality as possible.

I continued my task of visiting the few patients left in the department. I put on my most cheerful and uplifted face while making the rounds. Sometimes it helps to *pretend* like everything is fine when you know that the absolute worst is taking place in the other portion of the ER. Thankfully everyone was well-taken care-of and no one wanted for anything. I relegated myself back to my computer which was close to the closed trauma doors. I couldn't hear anything, but having lived that experience once, I knew the trauma that was being created in the minds of my young co-workers. Many had never been part of a paediatric code. I hurt for them and the family already, without being aware that at that moment, time of death was being called for the child.

I knew the instant that everything stopped. There was a shift in the air somehow. Everything and everyone grew quiet, which can only mean that the worst has happened.

The mother's wails wouldn't be contained by the tinted glass doors. The sound carried, and in my soul I cried too. The loss of another innocent child raked through every cell in my being. The memories of my first loss came flooding back. All I could do was put my head between my knees, shielded by the desk, as I let one sob escape my body. The torment radiating from the trauma room was overwhelming to say the least.

I allowed myself to have that moment of despair. I knew I needed to feel the pain in order to let it go easier later. I let myself feel the sadness, empathizing with the mother and her loss but then I knew I needed to support those who had been in the code and who now had their own trauma to contend with. I decided that it was my job to also care for those who had been inside the room so they could return and care for the patients that still needed them. The death of a child is an unbelievable trauma to witness and then be forced to act like nothing happened for the final hours of shift.

I made sure again that my patients were taken care of before turning my concern to the caregivers themselves. I got water, tissues, hot blankets and rounded up some snacks. I made sure that if anyone wanted or needed a hug, that they got it as they left the trauma room one by one. Those with young children at home seemed to need a little space, while others were quick to accept the hugs and someone to look after them for a minute.

The overnight doctor was someone I knew would take the loss personally. We separated him into the doctor's lounge, set him up with some food, a warm blanket and turned off the lights. He didn't look like himself, clearly haunted by the child he was unable to save. We left him, as he continued to say he was fine and weakly fought off our help. I knew he needed time to process. As we closed the door, I saw him crumble. His head slipped into his hands and his body folded forwards as he slid off the couch. I knew the sobs were coming so I quickly closed the door before anyone else could hear.

I took inventory of where everyone was. Some were sitting at their desks staring absently at their computer screen. Some were texting "tell the kids I love them" to spouses. Some were in the bathroom, taking a moment to prepare themselves to face their remaining patients. I continued to run between nurses, my doctor, and the residents, trying my best to make sure everyone was taken care of. We cried together, we hugged, and some were a little standoffish, but I understood it all. The benefit of figuring out I was an empath was that I could feel where everyone was sitting emotionally, which helped me to give them what they needed.

It was easily an hour or two before the coroner had come and gone, giving us the "all clear" to prepare the child for the morgue. My charge nurse took it upon herself to get everything ready, sparing others from having to do any more of the traumatizing work. This was one of a few small lifeless bodies that she had wrapped during her long career. She prepared the small body for the morgue and arranged for the security team to bring down the morgue stretcher without many of us noticing, because as we sat at our desks— in the wee early hours of the morning— all the power shut off in the department.

The department was completely *silent* as we were submerged in darkness. This had never happened before and it took everyone by surprise. No one said a word, staying completely still for a protracted 2-3 minutes. Imagine, an *entire* emergency department still and silent, knowing there was a recent death in the department—a department that very rarely saw death within its four walls. I felt a shiver run though me, a feeling of being unwell and very unhappy. At the time I didn't think anything of it but looking back, I think it was the spirit of the child.

When the lights finally came back on, they were only at half power. The back-up generator had kicked in but only things plugged into the emergency outlets were running. So now, what was usually a bright, loud, happening kind of department (even overnight) was operating on half power. Everyone started speaking softly because the lights were dimmed. All the background noise that we had become accustomed to had stopped. The water and ice machine stood silent in the corner. The comforting hum of the refrigerator and freezer in the other corner of the department was also missing. It seemed, as odd as it may sound, that the department was trying to grieve for the loss of the child.

The shift continued despite the obvious change in the air. Everything seemed a little off but we put on a brave face— until the lights shut off again only a few hours later.

Everyone tried to stay calm, stopping what they were doing and waiting. Within a few minutes the lights came on but again it was only the emergency lights casting light dimly throughout the halls. We were chatting amongst ourselves, when my charge nurse came up to our group, looking paler than I'd ever seen her. She stood there for a second, looking like she was going to say something, but remained silent.

"Are you alright?" I asked.

"I don't know," she said flatly.

"What happened?" I asked as gently as I could.

"You know how the lights went off?" she said hesitantly. "I was in the trauma room and the first time the lights went off was exactly when we moved the patient's body to the morgue stretcher," she said looking as if she was about to throw up.

Chills rippled down my body, starting at the top of my head, slowly working their way down the back of my neck and arms. Goosebumps also popped up on my forearms, the little hairs on the back of my neck starting to stand up.

"That›s not the worst part," she said. "The same paramedic crew that originally brought the child in just brought someone else in," she said, looking paler still. "They asked how things went with the patient they had brought in before," her words getting smaller as she spoke. "When I said that the patient died," she paused. "All the lights went off again."

We all stood there dumbfounded. In the back of my head my thought was "the spirit is *not* happy." We didn't move, staring at her as she stared at the floor. It took several moments before we all stepped away. We never talked about that night again to each other, but I still often think about it.

Now, here is my "most told" story

I was just coming onto the ER dayshift. I'd had a beautiful drive in— the sun was shining, and it was a nice warm day. I had everything ready.

30 | MY BEST STORY

My bag and lunch were packed, and I was ready for a great day.

It was oddly quiet as I walked through the double doors into my department. (For those of you who have worked in an ER, you know you never actually say "quiet," you just refer to it as the q-word because it usually means something is about to go down.) I noticed that everybody was talking in hushed tones and were leaning in closely towards each another. I hear little chuckles and I'm wondering what in the world is going on. I went to the front of the department to see where I'm scheduled and find I'm assigned to the quick treatment area. I started looking for the nurse I was supposed to take a report from, but couldn't find her anywhere. I finally went to the back hall, and asked where she was.

"Oh," they chuckled. "She's in resuscitation." I knew something was up because they couldn't quite make eye contact with me.

I walk to the resuscitation area and again there's not a lot going on which is odd. Normally, there is talking and laughter, especially with shift change. There was only one bay in resuscitation that had the drapes pulled, so I call out for the nurse I'm looking for.

"Yeah. I'm here," she says. "But I'm busy. Do you want to report?"

I said, "No it's okay, I can wait in the back."

She sounded out of breath as she spoke. I hear a grunt and somebody else making gasping noises. At this point I'm worried that they need help, so I pop my head in and receive a visual that I *will never* forget.

I see two nurses, both gowned in yellow PPE with masks and gloves. Each nurse is holding the very large leg of a patient. In the middle, between the two nurses, is my doctor also gowned up in yellow PPE. He has his hand up to the elbow in this large patients' rectum. Granted, the doctor is of a smaller stature, but he literally had his arm up to his elbow in this person's behind.

All I could manage was, "Sorry, I didn't realize you were so busy. Ugghhh...are you guys, okay?"

"Oh yeah, I'm just grand," My doc piped up.

Now I understood why everybody was whispering. I found out later that I'd stumbled into the medical team's second or third attempt to get the object out of that patient's rectum. Apparently, the same patient had visited the ER with a similar issue in the past but they'd always been able to retrieve whatever object had been inserted. This time it was a different story.

Don't get me wrong, we understand embarrassing situations. Generally, nobody wants to admit what truly happened, but I can promise you we've either seen it before, or have had a similar situation. The triage nurse in the ER does not care what you put where. All we need to know is what it is what we're dealing with and how long it's been in place. That's it. There's no judgement, there's no questioning "why" because we all know why. We just want you to be safe.

The morning went on and I eventually got report and started work. It wasn't until much later that morning that out of nowhere, a short woman (who I learned was the patient's wife) came past my desk yelling "it's out" with no context. A few patients' give her a look, wondering what it was all about. Of course, all the nurses in the department knew exactly what she was referring to.

I heard later that the retrieval ended up being a food item. When the patient was alert and ready for discharge, the person doing discharge education asked why they would insert a food item into their rectum instead of a proper sex toy with a solid base to it?

The patient responded, "It was organic. I thought it would be better for me."

31 | EMOTIONAL RESILIENCE

RESILIENCE IS DEFINED AS "the ability to 'rebound' from adversity when one's ability to function has been to some degree impaired."[2] It's become the new nursing buzz word—everyone is talking about building resilience, how to find resilience and how to increase resilience. Alongside the term resilience also comes the notion of emotional intelligence. Emotional intelligence "forms an important part of nurses' clinical practice. Through emotional intelligence, nurses learn how to deal with their feelings, as well as provide emotional support to patients and their families in multi-dimensional clinical environments."[3]

Here are ways to build your resilience—if you even want to call it that. How about we say it's building your ability to deal with the insanity that is nursing?

Tips to building emotional resilience

1. *Take time to just be with yourself.* Learn to sit with your discomfort and feel your feelings.
   Numbing with substances (alcohol, food, drugs, sex, phone addiction) can only get you so far, for so long. Sometimes the best thing you can do is allow yourself to feel. It's okay to be vulnerable and let it all go: yell, shout, scream, cry. Just feel. We're good at building walls around ourselves. Unfortunately, walls don't allow us to *feel*. It will take time to heal from COVID-19 and other traumas that we've chosen not to acknowledge. COVID just made us all realize how close to the edge we really were.

2. *Engage in self-care.* Take time off if you can. If you can't say no to the begging or pleading that may be on the other end of the phone call to come in to work, then don't answer the phone. If you need to take a mental health break from nursing, do it! If you're not taking care of yourself how can anyone expect you to take care of others?

3. *Make plans with a friend.* Get out of the hospital and get out of your house. Go somewhere you've never been before. Talk about anything *other* than work and the news. Remember to nurture the topics and hobbies that fill you with joy.

4. *Make time for gratitude.* A gratitude journal can be an amazing tool. Try to write just one line, each morning or night. What are you grateful for at the start or end of a day? Your answers can be anything, no matter how small. Want to up the ante? Add what went well in the day or something you accomplished that you are proud of.

5. *Give yourself the grace of time.* This is not a weekend, one and done kind of healing. This will be an ongoing process where you have to make the effort to choose to participate in your own healing. You are not a victim. This is not happening *to you*; it's happening *for you*. We've put off our own healing for too long to have this only be about COVID. It's time to start healing ourselves.

6. *Get professional help if you need it.* Let's be honest, we all need professional help. Look into your benefits and determine if you have access to funding for counselling. Ask for referrals from colleagues. Do your own search. *Trust your gut* when reading about a councillor/therapist and the areas they specialize in. Then, (the hardest part) reach out. Make an appointment and *show up*. Show up for you. You deserve it. You deserve to feel happy again. Don't let fear prevent you from going. Therapy a no-judgement area with someone who is 100% there for you. Take the shot, do this for you.

7. *See your healthcare professional.* When was the last time you had a physical or a pap smear? It's time to do all the things that you've been putting off. See your doctor, Nurse Practitioner, holistic practitioner and *talk* about what you're going through. There may be underlying health conditions that are holding you back from feeling your best. It's one other person who is there to help and support you without judgement.

31 | EMOTIONAL RESILIENCE

8. *Get outside.* Go for a walk and take the opportunity to breathe deeply and listen to the nature around you. Take off your socks and shoes and walk in the grass (no poison ivy!). Feel the texture. Feel the cool sensation of the earth under your feet. Feel the early morning dew in between your toes. Soak it up. Soak up that vitamin D but don't forget your sunscreen.

9. *Watch that favorite movie, listen to that favorite song.* Do things that remind you of a simpler and easier time! Relive memories that have nothing to do with the current situations of your life. Go for a drive and feel the wind on your face. Let it take away your worries. Listen to music and *belt out* the words as you sing along. As the words leave your mouth, exhale all the bullshit along with it.

10. *Get moving!* Start thinking about exercise as a medication. It's proven to help with mood as it releases endorphins that help you feel better. Focus on the feeling you get after you go for a walk or run. I call myself "non-compliant" when I slack on the exercise, and it helps me make it more of an ongoing practice than a short-term solution.

11. *Eat what you want, but in moderation.* When the pandemic started, I gave myself *full* permission to eat whatever I wanted, whenever I wanted. While this felt like a good idea in the moment, the pounds I gained have made things less comfortable. Instead, I am choosing to eat what I want, but in smaller portions. I don't obsess or worry about the weight gain but it makes me mindful of how much I'm cramming into my mouth.

12. *Sleep.* Sleep when you can, where you can. Start making decisions around how much sleep you get. A sleep routine can help you wind down after a busy shift. If you're like me and can't get your mind to stop spinning, try guided mediations. It provides focus on things other than your to-do list. It purposefully slows you down and after a few days of practice, I promise you'll start to fall asleep faster. If staying asleep is your issue, you can always supplement with melatonin, available over the counter or talk to your medical professional about sleep aids. Many, many nurses use sleep aids so don't feel like you're the odd one out doing this.

These basic things will get you started along the road of building emotional resilience. It's an ongoing process, with good and bad days, but everything balances out in the end.

It's time to take care of you for a change!

JOURNAL PROMPT

What are your next steps to care for yourself?
_____
_____
_____
_____
_____
_____
_____
_____
_____

32 | AN ENDING OR A BEGINNING?

I TRULY BELIEVE THAT everybody has the ability to be intuitive and understand what they are feeling. Gaining an understanding of how someone *else* is feeling and how to use it to better your patient care is a game changer. It's time to tune in to the moments that make you uncomfortable and listen to the voice in your head that says there's something more going on. Feel what you're feeling in that moment. It's time to focus on ourselves instead of others. It may sound selfish, but I promise that it's a way to help people too.

Work will always be there. People get sick and need nursing care, but if you don't start putting yourself first, you may not be there to provide it. Would you leave a patient not showered for days? Would you forget to brush their teeth, or leave them in dirty clothes without proper food? Emotional pain is as damaging as physical pain and, if nothing else, this book expresses my hope that you will realize you are worthy of giving yourself time and attention. You're still a good nurse even if you don't overwork yourself to the point of burnout or hating the profession. Give yourself permission to look inward and give yourself a chance to heal. The next step is up to you. Do you keep with the status quo or are you going to make a different choice? It's time to start healing. Choose YOU this time.

If you're looking for a sign, this is it.

APPENDIX | MY ER PUMP-UP PLAYLIST

Music has always gotten me through whatever moment I need to get through. My ER pump up playlist is overused, yet still does the job. When the music comes on, I know that someone else is feeling exactly as I do even though we've never met. Enjoy!

- Baby Did a Bad Thing – Chris Issak
- Me Too – Meghan Trainor
- ...Ready For it? – Taylor Swift
- Freak (feat. Steve Bays) – Steve Aoki, Diplo & Deorro
- Stronger – Britney Spears
- Five Hours – Deorro
- Timber – (feat. Ke$ha) Pitbull
- Take it Off – Ke$ha
- Boss Bitch – Doja Cat
- Feal the Beat – Darude
- Go Hard (La.La.La) – Kreayshawn
- The Spook – KSHMR, Basskillers & B3nte
- My Own Worst Enemy – Lit
- Ready to go – Republica
- Stutter – Marianas Trench
- Freedom! – George Michael
- Cry for you – September
- Help – Lucky Rose & Jason Walker
- Save My Life (feat. Lovespeake) – David Guetta & MORTEN

- Levels – Avicii
- Ghosts 'n' Stuff (feat. Rob Swire) – Deadmau5
- Earth Song – Michael Jackson
- Boom – P.O.D.
- I Am (Feat. Flo Milli) – Yung Baby Tate
- Ashes – Stellar
- Popular Monster – Falling In Reverse
- Trouble's Coming – Royal Blood
- Shots (feat. LMFAO) – Lil Jon
- Party Like a Rock Star – Shop Boyz
- Butterfly – Crazy Town
- Party Up – DMX
- Dirrty (feat. Redman) – Christina Aguilera
- Never Again – Sofiya Grinko
- Blow – Ke$ha
- Venom – Eminem
- London Bridge - Fergie
- My Songs Know What You Did In The Dark (Light Em Up) – Fall Out Boy

What songs did I miss? What is your go to *jam*?

_____
_____
_____
_____
_____

GLOSSARY

C. Diff – Clostridium Difficile: a pathogen giving the poor host uncontrollable liquid diarrhea.

CPAP – Continuous Positive Airway Pressure: an airway intervention to help push out fluid in people's lungs. Usually used in congestive heart failure patients when they're fluid overloaded.

CPR – Cardiopulmonary Resuscitation

EMS – Emergency Medical Services (paramedics)

ER – Emergency Room

ET Tube – endotracheal tube: used in intubation. Usually has 10 ml balloon at the end to keep in place.

ICU – Intensive Care Unit

IO – Intraosseous

IV – Intravenous

Lipase – enzyme made in the pancreas that if elevated usually indicates pancreatitis.

NICU – Neonatal Intensive Care Unit

OR – Operating room

PACU – Post Anesthetic Recovery Unit or Recovery Room

PPE – Personal Protective Equipment

PRN – As needed medication

Rhabdomyolysis – severe muscle breakdown usually related to working out heavily or muscle breakdown from laying on the floor for hours.

RN – Registered Nurse: usually a four-year undergraduate program at a university (in Canada)

RPN – Registered Practical Nurse: graduate of a two-year college diploma program (in Canada)

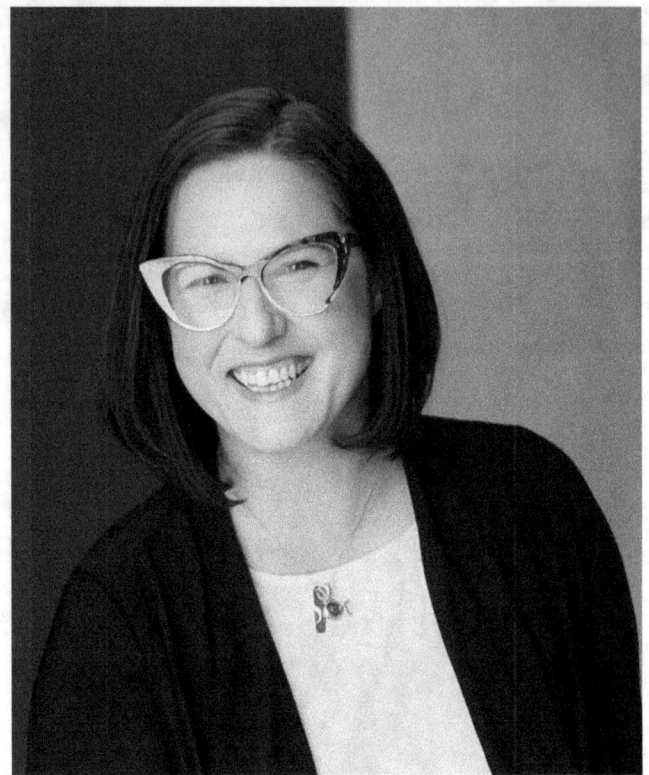

Jennifer Johnson is a wife, mother of two, and dedicated Registered Nurse based in Ontario, Canada. With sixteen years of experience working in emergency rooms across northern and southern Ontario, she has witnessed the heartbreak, drama, bullying, and life-or-death moments that define ER nursing. Her career, marked by resilience and compassion, took a profound turn during the pandemic—a time that tested not only her skills, but also her spirit.

ENDNOTES

1. Griffin, M. (2004). Teaching cognitive rehearsal as a shield for lateral violence: An intervention for newly licensed nurses. *The Journal of Continuing Education in Nursing, 35*(6), 257–263. https://doi.org/10.3928/0022-0124-20041101-07
2. Woodruff, R. A. (2018). The Eustress Experience of Registered Nurses: A Grounded Theory Study. Retrieved July 16, 2021, from https://www.proquest.com/openview/c7a5b5835ee241e7d2be0b4f-58382cb1/1?pq-origsite=gscholar&cbl=18750.
3. Abdi, A., Hassani, P., Jalali, R., & Salari, N. (2016). Use of intuition by critical care nurses: A phenomenological study. *Advances in Medical Education and Practice,* 65. https://doi.org/10.2147/amep.s100324

www.ingramcontent.com/pod-product-compliance
Lightning Source LLC
LaVergne TN
LVHW011829060526
838200LV00053B/3946